# HONEY
# SAPIENS

## Human cognition and sugars – the ugly, the bad and the good

### Mike McInnes MRPS

With a foreword by Fred Provenza,
Emeritus Professor of Behavioural Ecology

BOOKS

Hammersmith Health Books
London, UK

First published in 2023 by Hammersmith Health Books
– an imprint of Hammersmith Books Limited
4/4A Bloomsbury Square, London WC1A 2RP, UK
www.hammersmithbooks.co.uk

**Disclaimer:** This book is designed to provide helpful information on the
subjects discussed. It is not meant to be used, nor should it be used, to diagnose
or treat any medical condition. For diagnosis or treatment of any medical
problem, consult your own physician or healthcare provider. The publisher
and author are not responsible for any specific health or allergy needs that may
require medical supervision and are not liable for any damages or negative
consequences from any treatment, action, application or preparation, to any
person reading or following the information in this book. References are
provided for informational purposes only and do not constitute endorsement of
any websites or other sources. Readers should be aware that the websites listed
in this book may change. The information and references included are up to
date at the time of writing but given that medical evidence progresses, it may
not be up to date at the time of reading.

British Library Cataloguing in Publication Data: A CIP record of this book is
available from the British Library.

Print ISBN 978-1-78161-221-7
Ebook ISBN 978-1-78161-222-4

Commissioning editor: Georgina Bentliff
Typeset by: Julie Bennett of Bespoke Publishing, UK
Cover design by: Madeline Meckiffe
Cover image by: Shutterstock/Stmool/Nikita Chisnikov/Dernkadel
Index by: Dr Laurence Errington
Production: Deborah Wehner of Moatvale Press Ltd
Printed and bound by: TJ Books, Cornwall, UK

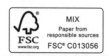

MIX
Paper from
responsible sources
FSC
www.fsc.org    FSC® C013056

# Contents

This book is dedicated to my grandchildren –
Oskar, Rob, Isla, Aaron and Huey.

# Foreword

Researchers believe honeybees evolved from carnivorous wasps and that pollen-feeding, called 'pollinivory', allowed bees to rapidly evolve and diversify. For over 100 million years, honeybees have been co-evolving with flowering plants. The honey they make from nectar-producing flowers is rich in energy and a host of phytochemicals that bees use to nourish and self-medicate.

The waggle dance honeybees perform provides details for other bees of the location, distance, and quality of pollen sources. Aristotle observed the waggle dance and noted bees returned to the same flowers. In 1973, Austrian biologist Karl von Frisch won a Nobel Prize for translating the dance's meaning. Young bees learn how to do these dances from experienced bees. Sadly, today there's a threat to the dance. Widely used pesticides can harm the honeybees' ability to learn. After exposure to toxins, the waggle dance changes. Bees make more errors.

In response to fungal infections, honeybees immunize their hives by foraging for plant resins (phenolics and terpenes), a behavior termed '*social immunity*'. Their colony-level use of resins lessens the need for chronic elevation of an individual bee's immune response. Bees' needs for more diverse diets to maintain colony health is gaining increasing appreciation. Yet, despite low phytochemical diversity, 1.6 million colonies are annually put in monocultures of almond orchards in California, and that's reducing the life expectancy of bees. Bees experience nutritional deficits when foraging on a single pollen source, and the lack of phenolics, terpenes, and other phytochemicals is adversely affecting social immunity. Phytochemically-rich diets enhance nutrition, reduce loads of parasites and enhance detoxification of pesticides.

Compared to honeybees, humans (*Homo sapiens*) have lived on Earth a very short time – roughly 300,000 years. During most of that time, our ancestors were hunters and gatherers who used animals of all sorts, including bees and honey, and hundreds of plants, for food, medicine, clothing and shelter. Only in the past 10,000 years did we transition from hunters and gatherers to pastoralists and small-scale farmers. And only during the past century did we create civilizations reliant on fossil fuels and industrial agriculture. In the process, we transformed from sunlight-driven ecological economies linked with the landscapes that nourish and sustain us to capitalist economies disconnected from nature and utterly dependent upon fossil fuels.

Fossil-fuel based agriculture enabled the food industry to mass-produce ultra-processed foods. These 'foods' link artificial flavors with metabolically mediated feedback from cells and organ systems in response to energy-rich compounds such as fructose and glucose, that together obscure nutritional sameness and can destroy health. The levels of ultra-processed foods now in our diet are an unprecedented recent phenomenon, but their effects are impossible to ignore.

According to the World Health Organization, and as this book sets out, around two billion humans are overweight or obese and 500 million are diabetic. Dementia, including its most common cause, Alzheimer's disease, accounts for a further 100 million humans, while autism spectrum disorders are thought to affect around 140 million humans. Thus, the total number of humans expressing sugar-driven neurodegeneration is around 2.67 billion globally, or one third of the global population.

These figures have risen markedly since the 1970s, changes

that coincide with a shift in diets away from fat to carbohydrates. That occurred as scientists such as Ancel Keys and politicians in the US, such as George McGovern, argued dietary fat elevated levels of cholesterol and caused cardiovascular disease. That was codified in nutrition guidelines that favored carbohydrates over fats. That's when fat became toxic and 'fat-free' came to dominate the shelves of grocery stores as the food industry rolled out a surfeit of '"foods" high in refined carbohydrates and sugar.

During a meal, refined carbohydrates and sugar quickly break down to glucose that fuels the neurons in the brain. Though the brain is only 2% of the human body by weight, it uses 20% to 25% of the energy a person consumes. To meet their needs, neurons require a fuel high in energy, but to prevent toxic excesses or devastating deficits, their regulatory mechanisms must be highly sophisticated. Neurons can function on ketones derived from fat, but their preferred fuel is glucose. Muscles, too, can function on ketones, but for activities that require much energy, they need glucose. Thus, the brain and muscles can, during times of great need, compete for glucose.

In *Honey Sapiens*, pharmacist Mike McInnes develops an integrative hypothesis for the upstream neurological cause of obesity, type 2 diabetes, Alzheimer's disease and autism. He begins by describing the brain as an internal combustion engine. He highlights the relationship between fuel (glucose), the fuel pump (glutamine synthetase) and the fuel governor (insulin). Oxidative stress occurs when excess intake of refined carbohydrates and sugars are quickly converted to glucose, which suppresses glutamine synthetase. That deprives neurons in the brain of the energy they require to live. Insulin resistance by cells throughout the body causes the pancreas to over-secrete insulin (hyperinsulinaemia). Hyperinsulinaemia exacerbates the challenge of excess circulating glucose (hyperglycaemia) by regulating and suppressing glutamine synthetase. This creates a toxic cycle: excess glucose inhibits glutamine synthetase and deprives neurons of the energy they require. The hunger that accompanies hyperinsulinaemia causes overeating, and obesity that so often precedes diabetes, as the brain attempts in vain to nourish itself.

Based on this hypothesis, Mike maintains that excessive weight and obesity are neurodegenerative diseases, characterised by diversion of glucose/energy from the brain where it is needed into the body where it is converted to fat and stored. He uses the term 'neurodegenerative' because overweight/obesity causes chronic energy deprivation of the human brain, loss of neurons, and brain shrinkage. Diabetes is a similar condition in which excess circulating glucose/energy can no longer be controlled by conversion to fat, and blood concentration rises to dangerous levels (hyperglycaemia). Autism, too, is a neurodegenerative disease but one that occurs due to excess sugar-induced teratogenesis (toxicity-driven malformation) during fetal development.

Yet, Mike argues, carbohydrates played a key role in the evolution of the human brain. This may seem paradoxical, as he also argues that over-consumption of ultra-processed foods high in refined carbohydrates and sugar that quickly digest to glucose, influences obesity, type 2 diabetes, Alzheimer's disease, autism, and the rapid decline in cognition, communication and language characteristic of the last 50 years. To explain that apparent paradox, we return to the honeybee.

Honeybees nourish themselves with honey, which is about 40% fructose, 30% glucose and 17% water, with the remainder being other sugars, carbohydrates, vitamins and minerals. A tablespoon of honey provides about 4600 calories of energy. An ounce (28 grams) of honey would fuel a bee's flight around the world. On this high-energy diet, a honeybee can fly up to 15 miles per hour, while their wings beat about 11,400 times per minute. A bee in flight seeking forage increases its metabolic rate 70 times, and yet its brain is protected from neurotoxicity.

# Foreword

Unlike a modern human, a honeybee knows how to fuel its brain with sugars and at the same time protect its body from harm. How does a honeybee do that without damaging its nervous system? Bioflavonoids in pollen and honey protect bees' brains from oxidation and inflammation. Bioflavonoids, which are much older than honeybees or flowering plants, arose some 3.5 billion years ago, a time when the first blue-green algae appeared on earth. Blue-green algae are among the earliest organisms to create energy from sunlight via photosynthesis.

Photosynthesis and protective bioflavonoid antioxidants are biological twins that benefit plants, bees, and humans. Our hunter-gatherer ancestors knew honey protected health and improved cognition. They knew honeybees were the source of this nourishment, and they learned to harness this fuel without harming the life cycle of bees. Rock art in Spain, India, Southern Africa and Australia portrays honeybees and honey hunting late in the Paleolithic period from 40,000 to 8000 years ago. These artistic renditions depict a vitally important facet of human evolution, and many studies show the key role of honey in the diets of extant hunter-gatherers.

Mike concludes this book with a hypothesis. Genetic analyses show the gene that expresses the salivary enzyme amylase, which digests starch to glucose in the mouth and stomach, is 600,000 years old. Thus, our ancestors were eating starchy roots and tubers early in our evolution, long before the advent of farming 10,000 years ago. This is the time in our evolutionary history when the brain expanded most rapidly. For humans, glucose is the primary fuel of the brain, and starchy foods provide glucose in abundance. This change in diet may have exerted a major evolutionary influence by providing the fuel that accelerated the growth of the brain. In addition to starchy roots and tubers, where might our ancestors have found a readily accessible, sustainable, storable and renewable source of energy that had its own regulatory properties and could catalyse the exponential growth and neurodevelopment of the human brain? Mike argues that, like honeybees, our evolution too was enabled by flowering plants through the pollen that is transformed by bees into the honey that fueled the expansion of our brain.

**Fred Provenza** BS MS PhD
Professor Emeritus, Department of Wildland Resources, Utah State University, USA

# About the Author

**Mike McInnes** is a pharmacist and sports nutritionist who has worked with many athletes. After selling his award-winning pharmacy business to Boots in 1997 he began researching the specifics of energy partition and selection in exercise and has continued to research the relationship between sugars and energy, especially for enhancing mental and sports performance, for over 20 years. He is the author of *The Honey Diet* (Hodder 2014, also translated into German) and *The Hibernation Diet* (2007).

# Acknowledgements

A very special thank you to my publisher and editor, Georgina Bentliff. I am lucky to have found (after countless efforts) a publisher/editor in the field of health/medical publishing such as Georgina, who was able to notice and appreciate what I was wanting to say and had the required vision, patience and knowledge to edit this book. From a sprawling and disjointed manuscript, Georgina battered, bullied and buffeted my offering into an organised and readable popular science text. I cannot thank Georgina enough.

I must also thank Emeritus Professor Fred Provenza of Utah State University who has written the Foreword to this book. He is an award-winning pioneer of plant, soil, animal and human nutrition. In his wonderful book *Nourishment*, he has shown how these are positively linked in the wild, and negatively in industrial agriculture. His team is instrumental in creating BEHAVE – committed to integrating behavioural principles and processes with local knowledge to enhance ecological, economic and social values of rural and urban communities and landscapes. There is no other nutritional expert internationally that I could have wished for to provide a Foreword for this book. I am profoundly grateful.

My friend Alex Dunedin is the Founder of the Ragged University, a wonderful educative institution that draws on knowledge from individuals (academic or other) willing to share their intellectual interests and passions with the wider

# Acknowledgements

community in cafes, pubs, art galleries and other public spaces. I have fruitfully discussed cerebral energy metabolism and its impairments, along with sugar, fat and protein metabolism, with Alex for 20 years over coffees and beers. Long may it continue.

I am grateful too to David Elliot, a business consultant with a deep knowledge of, and special interest in, nutrition, who over a period of more than a decade supported my research and provided many studies and links into sugar and honey metabolism that I had missed. Thank you, David.

# Editorial note

In this book you will encounter scientific names, some of which will not be new to you and some that will at first seem strange, and that are not usually discussed in the daily health discourses that occupy us. These include glial cells, oxidation, inflammation, glutamate, glutamine, glutamine synthetase, the glutamate/glutamine cycle and glutathione among many others. However, if you read this book, I can promise that these terms will become as familiar and as easy to understand as words like 'Prozac' and 'serotonin reuptake inhibitors' that were previously known only to physicians, pharmacists and health professionals, and are now as widely discussed as the latest film blockbuster or Netflix serial. To make this even easier, I have included a Glossary at the end to explain all of these and more.

You will also encounter a lot of scientific research that I have been curating for many years, some of it recent and some of it much older. This is all listed in a standard format, organised by chapter, starting on page 185. For many references I have included an interpretative note. These represent my views as the author of this book in the context of the *Honey Sapiens* hypothesis – that excess sugars are leading to neurodegeneration at every stage of human life. They are not necessarily the views of the study authors, who often have not recognised the remarkable implications of their findings.

*Honey Sapiens* is a book that seeks to open a discussion with the public that has, until now not been warned about the neurodegenerative results of excess consumption of refined sugars. I leave you, the reader, to review my arguments and the research and come to your own conclusions.

Finally, readers may find some repetition between chapters. This is an inevitable consequence of looking at the effects of excess dietary sugars as a whole, and also with regard to four different neurodegenerative conditions. The implications of research findings often apply to more than one condition and also have general application. I consequently offer no apology for repetition but would like to emphasise it is necessary and deliberate at times.

# Introduction

Dear Reader,

In this book I will show you that refined carbohydrates and sugars are shrinking the human brain and degrading human cognition. The conditions that express this cognitive apocalypse are obesity, type 2 diabetes, Alzheimer's disease (the most common cause of dementia) and autism spectrum disorders, and I will show that all are neurodegenerative conditions involving lack of energy to the brain. The mechanism that drives these ailments is that of excess circulating glucose which oxidises and degrades an enzyme that you may have never heard of but which is an essential part of the human brain's fuel pump; this is glutamine synthetase, the full importance of which I describe in Chapter 2. Excess circulating glucose suppresses this enzyme and thereby deprives the brain of energy, as would occur in any engine, mechanical or biological; overwhelming the engine disables the fuel pump.

*Excess sugar in the bloodstream deprives the brain of energy.*

The first condition for life is energy homeostasis, the balance between fuel income and output. The second is coupling environmental information with the energy required to navigate the environment consistent with survival. Homo sapiens is the only known animate species that is losing both these vital functions, and this is a quite recent development, correlated with the period when we altered our diet in favour of increased consumption of refined carbohydrates and sugars, over the last half century. The differing varieties of disease simply express the timing, degree and duration of the sugar assault on the provision of energy to the brain, before and after birth.

In obesity and diabetes, we see reduced cerebral volume and cognitive impairments; in Alzheimer's disease, reduced cerebral volume, cognitive decline and dementia. In autism spectrum disorders there are structural alterations in the brain and compromised cognition, communication and language as well as a range of other symptoms, including epilepsy and visual impairments. Everything else – each of the degenerative pathways and impaired mechanisms, the damaged enzymes, receptors and hormones, that pharmaceutical companies attempt to repair with synthetic drugs – are  *downstream, and therefore doomed to failure.*

## The only 'good' sugar – Honey

In this book I will also show that if we replace refined sugar with honey to sweeten our food and drink, we can prevent (though not treat) and ultimately reverse the catastrophic and unnecessary tragedy that is befalling human cognition. If that seems a tall order, it is not. In Chapter 9 I will show you that honey is the most extraordinary fuel ever produced. Furthermore, I will show that it is the perfect energy source for the brain, and that its neglect by the health institutions over the previous two decades, during which the science of this knowledge has grown exponentially, is both a tragedy and an intellectual crime.

The only possible solution is the removal of refined carbohydrates and sugars from foods and drinks. We can follow a diet without these altogether or we can replace them with honey. Honey is the most potent antidiabetic food known to us.[1] It is also emerging as a strong candidate for being the food/fuel that gave rise to the cognitively advanced brain of Homo sapiens and fostered the cognitive leap that created our species (see page 172). Sugars are damaging fuels; honey is a fuel that protects the human brain from sugar toxicity and at the same time upregulates the expression of genes that are key for communication.

The honeybee, unlike all other living species, has developed in honey its own fuelling system in coevolution with flowering plants over a period of 100 million years. Honey is richly endowed with an army of bioflavonoids (plant nutrients) that protect the enzyme glutamine synthetase from oxidative degeneration. If humans double the sugar load in their bloodstream, they become diabetic and are at risk of blindness, kidney loss, gangrene and compromised cognition. The honeybee carries in its circulation (known as haemolymph) not double, not 10 times, but 50 times the level of sugars carried by humans, without difficulty.[2] I will show that the honeybee brain, with its advanced cognitive abilities during foraging, is the most sublime model of how to fuel an energy-expensive engine (the brain) with combustible sugars and yet protect it from toxic sugar oxidative degradation.

## Sugar and the brain

Unless you are deliberately restricting your carb/sugar intake to force your brain and body to run on ketones ('keto-adapted' – see pages 27, 237), as you read this, your brain is burning a toxic fuel to do so – the sugar known as glucose. Glucose is the fuel of consciousness, thought, cognition, social communication and language. If for any reason its delivery into the brain were to be compromised, you would have difficulty knowing who you are, who you are related to and where you are, and you would thus have lost the survival knowledge that enables you to navigate the world that you live in. Does that remind you of any of the conditions I am going to be focusing on?

*The first condition of life is energy homeostasis – maintaining the balance between energy supply and demand.*

Only in special circumstances, such as during starvation or fasting or when eating a very low-carb diet, does the human brain burn other types of fuel, known as ketones. I describe in Chapter 5 how it has been shown to be possible to run the body healthily on ketones (page 80), but for most people on the planet, and almost everyone in the 'civilised' world', at any given moment, every one of the 100 billion cells that comprise their brain is powered by glucose.

However, the human brain has no significant internal fuel store. This means it is reliant on a continuous supply of glucose every nanosecond of its life, and this is delivered by the bloodstream. A sudden fall in blood glucose concentration (known as hypoglycaemia) is catastrophic for the brain. If not quickly resolved, it will lead to confusion, loss of consciousness, coma and then death. If there were any doubt about the relationship between glucose and human cognition, hypoglycaemia perfectly confirms that link; if an individual with insulin-dependent diabetes misjudges the dose and injects too much insulin, which drives glucose out of the blood, a hypoglycaemic episode may lead to disaster.

*Our brains have no significant internal fuel store and must rely at all times on sufficient supplies in the bloodstream.*

This absolute reliance that most of us have on glucose

extends beyond the brain, which acts as the processing centre, and includes the spinal cord and the entire nervous system throughout the body – the system which carries impulses that control all the organs, tissues and glands, and transmits sensory information to muscles that coordinate our movement and locomotion. However, since we consider the brain to be the true origin of our thinking and communication, I focus almost exclusively on it in this book. This should not in any way exclude the feedback from the body to the brain; all organs, glands and tissues take part in this – for instance, the gut has a profound influence on all brain activity, including that of cognition via the vagus nerve. And all nerve cells rely on glutamine synthetase for their energy supply, not just those in the brain.

## Sugar can be dangerous

The human brain functions as an internal combustion engine (ICE) – that is, it consumes energy, creates heat and performs work. It is hungry, very hungry, and burns fuel at a colossal rate; a neurone (nerve cell) burns around 20 times more fuel than any other cell in the human body. Indeed, the human brain is one of the highest consumers of fuel in nature.[3] It burns up to 6.5 grams of glucose hourly – that is, 150 grams daily, one kilo weekly and 50 kilos annually (approximately 110 pounds or a hundredweight) of glucose. If it does not receive the fuel it needs it will rapidly cease to function. However, too much sugar can be equally disastrous.

If you doubt that sugar is a combustible fuel, the history of sugar production is one of major explosions at sugar refineries, the most recent being at Port Wentworth in Georgia USA, in 2008, with fatal consequences. Sugar dust is highly explosive. Indeed, so useful is sugar as a combustible fuel that in Brazil, a major cane-sugar-producing country, it has been developed into one of the major fuels that drive the nation's cars. The sugar is harvested and converted into alcohol, which translates the high-energy compound into a form that can be easily used by a normal engine with an added special device. By 2006 there were already 30,000 fuel stations that supplied automotive energy in this form, which is both highly efficient and cost effective. American auto-manufacturers are making such cars in Brazil, and the prospect of doing so in the USA, to avoid pollution, is becoming more and more attractive.

This means that sugar is a dangerously combustible fuel and needs to be carefully regulated. The body has developed a brilliant system for balancing its benefits with its dangers, but when those mechanisms are overwhelmed by excessive consumption of sugar, as I will show, neurodegeneration follows.

We have benefited enormously from sugar in the foods we consume, and we can credit this lovely, sweet-tasting food with powering Shakespeare's plays, Einstein's Theory of Relativity, Bach's Mass in B Minor, Robert Burn's *A Man's a Man for A' That*, Michelangelo's David, Picasso's Guernica, Tolstoy's *War and Peace* and the development of Apollo 11, among boundless other achievements that have emanated from human cognition, communication and language. However, from its long evolutionary history, over a miniscule period of 50 years, excess consumption has become the driving force of rapid decline of these faculties, the very faculties that define our species.

Humans have been enslaved by sugar; firstly expressed in the enslavement of African labourers who were captured and transported across the Atlantic to cut and process the sugar cane; secondly in our ongoing addiction to sugar; thirdly in the neurodegenerative conditions obesity, type 2 diabetes, Alzheimer's disease and autism spectrum disorders; and fourthly in the corruption of the intellectual capital of the health institutions that has facilitated and resulted in these conditions. I describe these enslavements in greater detail in Chapter 2.

## In summary...

In this book I will show you, dear reader, that every time you add a spoonful of refined sugar to a cup of tea or coffee, you are digesting your brain – yes, digesting your cerebral organ and degrading your cognition. If, on the other hand, you add the same quantity of sugar in the form of honey, you are protecting your brain and enhancing your cognition. As you will discover, the choice is yours.

## Important note

While honey is the perfect sweetener in most cases it must NOT be given to children under 1 year old. This is because it contains bacteria which may include botulinum that a more mature gut can handle without a problem but a very young gut may have difficulties with. As it is better to keep babies and young children away from sweetened foods altogether so they do not develop a 'sweet tooth' with all the downstream problems discussed in this book, the exclusion of honey should not be an issue.

# Chapter 1

## Sugars – the ugly,
## the bad and the good

The first condition of life from the tiniest bacterium to the largest animal known, the blue whale, is energy homeostasis – that is, balancing energy income with output. Animate species that achieve this have existed for hundreds of million years. Our species, *Homo sapiens,* has existed for around 200,000 years and, until very recently, successfully did so. That success is now under threat from the very substances that bring life – sugar and oxygen.

Throughout this book I talk about 'sugars' and 'refined carbohydrates' but what all of these reduce down to is the simple sugars that form the building blocks of all the fibre, starches, carbohydrates and complex sugars that, along with fats and proteins, make up all living things. And when I talk about 'circulating sugar' or 'sugar in the bloodstream' it is glucose that is the issue – the simple sugar that our cells can use for energy but which, if supplied in overwhelming quantities, either in its simple form or in a more complex form that can be very quickly and easily broken down for use (e.g. in white bread or pasta), will disable the energy system that supplies our nervous system and leave our brains starving.

How was it that this small and very simple molecule (glucose) became the fuel that gave rise to conscious life some 3.8 billion years ago? And how did it come to be used by all animate species, including humans, for vision, hearing, thought and communication?

## Photosynthesis: Creating the fuel of life

Glucose is created as a result of a process known as photo-synthesis, by which plants and other green organisms convert radiant light energy from the sun into chemical energy. This energy is stored in the form of glucose, a simple 6-carbon molecule, synthesised from the gas carbon dioxide and water. Although this synthesis may seem quite simple, the process is infinitely complex, and science has not yet fully articulated the mechanisms. If and when we do so, we will be able to power civilisation directly from the sun, without the need for fossil fuels, nuclear power or other costly and environmentally toxic energy projects.

The glucose thus created can then be used to build a huge range of more complex molecules, including 'table sugar' or 'sucrose', which consists of glucose and fructose, another simple sugar made by photosynthesis as a secondary product. These 'mono' (single) saccharides (sugars) and 'di' (two (such as sucrose)) saccharides can then come together as 'poly' (many) saccharides which can form the fibre that gives plants their structure and starches, that are an efficient way to store sugar/ energy, for example in root vegetables. Just as these complex molecules can be built up, so can they be broken down again to their simplest forms. In living organisms enzymes, most of which are highly specific, do that. For example, amylase breaks down sucrose to fructose and glucose in our mouths and stomachs.

But it all starts with photosynthesis, without which none of these biochemicals could exist and there would be no life.

## Understanding sugars, starches and carbohydrates

As I've said, the key 'sugar' in this book is glucose as that is what we humans use as fuel, but so that you can understand how you might be overwhelming your body – and brain – with sugar without apparently consuming large quantities of what you think of as sugar I am including a very brief description of what is involved.

Humans can digest many polysaccharides – though not insoluble fibre, which has other benefits including for our digestive health. However, we cannot absorb these polysaccharides until we have broken them down to their most basic form. Fructose (often called 'fruit sugar') is, perhaps surprisingly, easier to absorb than glucose; it travels across the walls of our small intestine without any energy expenditure or the need for sodium. However, fructose can be used in the human body only in the liver, where it is broken down and rebuilt into the polysaccharide, glycogen. This is a storage sugar, ready and waiting for use by the brain when blood sugar runs low. However, as we will learn, when glycogen is called out of storage (now as glucose) because the brain is in need of energy, it can only do its job with the help of the enzyme glutamine synthetase, the fundamental and essential enzyme that is the star of this book.

Our human cells have the wonderful ability to run on two fuels – either glucose or ketones – which has made us highly adaptable to different climates and environments and sources of nutrition. If given a choice, however, their first choice is glucose. (An interesting point to note here is that cancer cells can run only on glucose, not ketones, but that is not the focus of this book.)

Glucose travels across the intestinal wall with the help of a specific transport protein that requires dedicated energy and the presence of sodium, its co-transport partner. It then travels through the intestinal bloodstream via the liver, and on to the general bloodstream to feed all the cells in the body and brain. Excess glucose can also be stored in the liver as glycogen.

All complex carbohydrates (polysaccharides) thus have to be broken down if we are to use them for energy. The speed with which our digestive processes can do this and thereby get the constituent simple sugars into the bloodstream, varies according to many other factors, including the type of polysaccharide, the presence of fibre, the presence of micronutrients (minerals, vitamins, plant chemicals etc) that can enable or inhibit digestion and absorption, and the co-presence of the other macronutrients, fats and proteins. This is all highly complex but the important issue to be aware of is that if you eat a bowl of white rice your body can turn it into glucose almost as quickly as if you had eaten the same amount of calories as table sugar. And the chances are you can eat a lot more rice than you would sugar, enough to overwhelm your brain's vital energy pump very quickly.

## The challenge facing Homo sapiens

The human brain is one of the highest consumers of energy in nature. It constitutes around 2% of the human body by weight, but accounts for 20–25% of all the energy consumed. For the delicate brain to process these quantities of combustible fuel, its regulatory mechanisms must be highly sophisticated, and the fuel source rich in energy-regulating principles – requirements fulfilled only by honey as I will show in Chapter 9. As I will describe in Chapter 3, overabundance of sugar has not been a feature of our evolutionary history, which may explain why we do not have an in-built regulatory system to deal with too much sugar. The levels of refined carbohydrates and sugars we are now seeing in our diet are an unprecedented and very recent phenomenon, but their effects are impossible to ignore.

*The total number of humans expressing sugar-driven neurodegeneration is around 2.67 billion globally – that is, one third of the global population.*

According to the World Health Organization (WHO), around two billion humans are overweight or obese.[1] Overweight and obesity are neurodegenerative diseases, characterised as they are by diversion of glucose/energy from the brain where it is needed

4

into the body where it is converted to fat and stored. I use the term 'neurodegenerative' because overweight/obesity causes chronic energy deprivation of the human brain, loss of neurones and brain shrinkage. As described in Chapter 6, type 2 diabetes is a similar condition in which excess circulating glucose/energy can no longer be controlled by conversion to fat, and blood concentration rises to dangerous levels (hyperglycaemia). There are an estimated 500 million humans worldwide who are diabetic. Dementia, including its most common cause, Alzheimer's disease, accounts for a further 100 million humans, while autism spectrum disorders are thought to affect around 2% of the world's population – that is, 140 million people. As I will explain later in this book, it too is a neurodegenerative disease but one that occurs due to sugar-induced teratogenesis (toxicity-driven malformation) during foetal development. This means the total number of humans expressing sugar-driven neurodegeneration is around 2.67 billion globally – that is, one third of the global population. These figures have risen disproportionately since the 1970s. What could be driving this very recent increase?

## Genetics versus environment

As I describe in this book, four neurodegenerative conditions have come to affect more than one third of the human population since the 1970s, and their incidences have dramatically increased in parallel, posing the fundamental question: What is the influence or influences behind these increases?

One of the more witless terms used by the health authorities to explain these neurodegenerative diseases is that of 'heterogeneity'. By heterogeneity they mean that there are so many different causes that it is impossible to identify any one as a principal cause. This is a neat way to avoid referencing dietary sugars as a primary influence, even though the incidence of each of these conditions increased dramatically in parallel with increased consumption of refined carbohydrates and sugars, from the 1970s on.

Of course, there are potentially many factors that may contribute to the increase in these conditions, such as genetic and epigenetic mechanisms and environmental toxins, including heavy metals, pesticides, herbicides and air pollution. However, none of these factors is universal and global. Overconsumption of refined sugars is universal and global.

Furthermore, the timing of these influences is itself a factor in causation; exposure to any environmental hazard depends for its outcome on the timing of that event in the life cycle of any individual – the earlier the exposure, the more dramatic is the likely effect on any organism. In humans, exposure of the embryo/foetus to a drug will have a significantly more damaging outcome compared to after birth. Autism and Alzheimer's disease share similar declines in cognition, communication and language, although each is expressed at opposite ends of the life cycle in humans.

## Genetic factors

Each of the conditions I address involves genetic input; indeed, it could not be otherwise. Every aspect of life and behaviour, be it physical, neurological or psychological, and including health and medical conditions, involves activation of multiple genes and gene sequences. However, any medical condition that involves many different genes must have some environmental influence that orchestrates these genes, and that was not present prior to the development of the condition. Multiple genes do not spontaneously self-organise to cause ill-health in an evolutionarily short space of time. All four conditions under the spotlight here have been associated with multiple genes, and that number grows with every new piece of research.

Expression of those genes (that is, which ones actually manifest and make a difference) alters with every passing

*Figure 1: The rise in sugar consumption and the*
*'sugar sickness syndromes'*

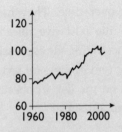

US sugar consumption 1960 to 2005
in lbs per year person[F1]

2023 = 126.4 g per day
(WHO recommends 25 g max)

**Obesity**
England[F2]

|      | 1975 | 5-10% of population |
|------|------|---------------------|
|      | 2018 | 25-30% of population |

USA[F3]

| 1950s | Men | 5.8% of population |
|-------|-----|---------------------|
|       | Women | 3.9% of population |
| 1990s | Men | 14.8% of population |
|       | Women | 14% of population |

**Type 2 diabetes**
Global[F4]       1990 = 18th leading cause of death
                 2017 = 9th leading cause of death

Global incidence  1980[F5] = 108 million
                  2014[F5] = 422 million
                  2017[F4] = 462 million
                  2021[F6] = 536.6 million (10.5%)
                  2045[F6] = 783.2 million (12.2%) predicted

**Alzheimer's disease**
Global[F7]       1990 = 20.3 million
                 2016 = 43.8 million
                 2050 = 152 million (predicted)

**Autism spectrum disorders (ASD)\***
USA[F8]          1980 = 1 in 10,000 8 year olds
                 2013 = 1 in 50 8 year olds
                 2018 = 1 in 44 (2.3%) 8 year olds
                 2023 = 1 in 36 (2.8%) 8 year olds

*Contributing factors for increase in ASD diagnosis: awareness,
change in diagnostic criteria (DSM-5), access to services AND
metabolic syndrome (insulin resistance/pre-diabetes)

moment of every passing day, depending on where we are, what we are doing and if we are sick or well. If the sugar sickness syndromes were genetically driven, their manifestation would remain within a quite small variation over time. They have, however, increased exponentially over the past five decades. Some major environmental factor is orchestrating the expression of these genes, and epigenetic influences (environmental factors that switch genes on and off) are high on the list, in obesity,[2] diabetes type 2,[3] Alzheimer's disease[4] and autism.[5]

## Epigenetics: The paradox of time

Time may influence health in a somewhat unexpected way, or perhaps relative time may be a more correct expression. Albert Einstein showed that time and space are interconnected, and that time is not a fixed or absolute dimension – that is, it may stretch or contract, depending on the speed of travel through space.[6] The faster we travel through space, the slower the time frame within which we travel. This has been dramatically shown in a recent experiment that involved identical twins and the influence of epigenetics.

Epigenetics is a branch of life science that involves changes to gene *expression* but not to underlying DNA that may influence health. For example, a person may have the gene for cystic fibrosis but it may not be expressed so they remain free of symptoms depending on environmental factors. These changes can be inherited – although the genes themselves remain unaltered, their expression is changed due to some environmental factor. Excess consumption of sugars is recognised as one such influence. There are many others. Identical twins share the same genes, but if separated at birth, the different environmental influences can result in different health and behavioural outcomes via epigenetic alterations that result in the expression of different genes.

In 2015, astronaut Scott Kelly travelled to the International Space Station, where he spent a year. His identical twin, Mark

Kelly, who was also a NASA astronaut, did not accompany him on that mission. This provided the space scientists with a perfect opportunity to study and compare the epigenetic effects on the same genetic profile, of space travel compared to residence on earth.

Perhaps not surprisingly, they found that there were major differences in health between the twins, not only physiologically and psychologically, but also in gene expression. One of the interesting alterations of gene expression in Scott was that the genes involved in the expression of the enzyme telomerase were affected, and that his telomeres (part of each cell's bundle of chromosomes) increased in length. The length of a telomere is an index of lifespan – the longer the telomere, the longer the lifespan.[7] Does this mean that space travel lengthens life, via time dilation?

Scott's telomeres returned to normal within two days of his return to Earth making it unlikely that the influence of Earth's gravity was involved; it seems that relativity of time was the key influence, as Einstein claimed, and that in this case the alteration of telomerase gene expression was epigenetically induced.

## Environmental factors

There are many potential environmental factors that may be involved in the rise of obesity, type 2 diabetes, Alzheimer's disease and autism spectrum disorders, from modern pesticides and herbicides to heavy metal and industrial toxin pollution, drugs, and so on that were not widespread before the 1970s and have become so after the post-WWII chemical revolution occurred. However, and as I have said, none of these is universal or global. The alteration in human diet, which began in the USA in the 1970s and rapidly spread around the world, and which substituted refined carbohydrates and sugars for fats in processed foods, *is* global and universal. It may be stated that this dramatic change in human diet has been the most significant alteration in the evolutionary history of our species. Since this was initiated and presided over by the leading health institutions in the world – namely, the National Institutes of Health in the United States of America and its equivalents in other countries, supported by governments and the powerful food and sugar lobbies – any attempt to raise a public discussion around the role of sugars has been ruthlessly suppressed.

Even today, when the role of excess consumption of sugars in the spread of ill health has emerged into the public domain, and sugar taxes have been introduced in some countries, any suggestion that this may be a significant factor in the explosive growth of Alzheimer's disease and autism spectrum disorders is avoided. If a food that is new in human diet just might negatively alter the life and health of one third of the human population, such that they are impaired physically, psychologically and cognitively, and their lifespan reduced, would it not be appropriate to devote significant scientific resources to discovering if that food is involved and reducing consumption, if it is? No such investigation has occurred and the public are left confused.

## The metabolic (energy dysregulation) diseases

As I will repeat throughout this book, the first condition of all animate life is energy homeostasis (balance) such that energy income matches energy output. Both deficiency and excess of energy are lethal. Late-modern humans, from the 1970s on, have been faced with a food environment that increasingly consists of high-energy, low-nutrient foods. The results of this toxic combination may be viewed in every healthcare setting around the world, where patients gather in the (increasingly futile) hope that they may be offered a treatment that might relieve the many symptoms that blight their lives and the futures of their children and grandchildren. These symptoms – the symptoms and complications of metabolic diseases – make up what I call the 'sugar-sickness syndromes':

*Symptoms of sugar sickness syndrome one: Obesity*
High blood pressure
Related heart disease and stroke
Increased risk of type 2 diabetes
Some cancers
Digestive problems
Sleep apnoea
Osteoarthritis
Increased susceptibility to infections such as Covid-19
Fatigue
Sensory processing problems
Neurological problems including cognitive impairment.

*Symptoms of sugar-sickness syndrome two: Type 2 diabetes*
Cardiovascular problems, including stroke
Excess and frequent urination
Increased thirst
Increased repeated hunger
Fatigue
Blurred vision
Blindness
Kidney damage leading to kidney loss
Gangrene and limb loss
Poor wound healing – abscesses
Tingling in hands and feet – peripheral neuropathy
Neurological degenerative problems, including cognitive
    impairments.

*Symptoms of sugar-sickness syndrome three: Alzheimer's disease*
Memory loss and confusion
Shortened attention span
Problems of learning
Numerical problems and confusion
Problems of organised thinking

Problems coping with new situations
Inability to recognise family and friends
Inability to recognise foods, and disorganised eating
Advanced neurological and cognitive impairments.

*Symptoms of sugar-sickness syndrome zero: Autism spectrum disorders*
Impaired cognition, communication and language
Poor eye contact
Inability to empathise/lack of 'theory of mind'
Flapping hands and repeated gestures
Repeating phrases and babbling
Heightened sensitivity or sensory aversion
Sensory processing disorders
Obsessive interests
Inability to change
Reliance on routine
Epilepsy
Gastrointestinal disorders, including constipation and
    diarrhoea
Gross-motor problems, including uncoordinated gait, and
    difficulties with fine motor control.

You may note that among the multiple problems listed that cause so much distress to individuals and family members, neurodegeneration and cognitive impairments feature as a common denominator in all four conditions. How is it possible that our species, which developed advanced cognition, communication and language over a period of 200,000 years, the only species known to have made this gigantic evolutionary leap, could have allowed itself to decline physiologically, psychologically and cognitively in the miniscule timespan of 50 years? It is time to look at what I call the 'four sugar enslavements of humankind', the focus of the next chapter.

# Chapter 2

# The sugar sickness syndromes: How did we get here?

*Homo sapiens* is sick – sugar-sick. And we have never been sicker, physiologically, psychologically or cognitively. What I call the 'sugar sickness syndromes' affect more than one third of the human population, expressed in four metabolic (energy dysregulation) diseases: obesity, type 2 diabetes, Alzheimer's disease and autism spectrum disorders. According to the World Health Organization (WHO), obesity affects around 2 billion humans, type 2 diabetes around 500 million, dementias including Alzheimer's disease around 50 million and autism 150 million.[1] These are astonishing figures, which have grown exponentially in the half-century since the 1970s, and place an enormous burden on health services around the world. Such is the rapidity of the increased spending on healthcare in 'advanced' countries that other important infrastructure projects, including transport, housing, education and security, are lagging behind and consistently under-resourced.

As we saw in Chapter 1, each of these conditions is lifestyle generated and non-communicable, and therefore avoidable. The rapidity of increase must exclude genetic causation factors as these do not vary significantly over time. Of course and as I said in the previous chapter, genetic susceptibility does play a part, as is the case in every disease, but multiple genes do not spontaneously work together to create a chronic condition in any animate species; there is no known evolutionary history for this type of degenerative ailment to occur. Studies that implicate genes in environmentally induced diseases are of great intellectual interest, and certainly contribute to the understanding of how environmental and genetic conditions intersect, but they do *not* offer improved understanding of causation.

These sugar-driven conditions have been described as 'diseases of civilisation'. They arose historically as humans became more and more 'advanced' and settled – the transition from being hunter-gatherers to agricultural farming and the domestication of crops; increasing population growth and consumption of grains are recognised as major influences. The popular view of our Stone Age ancestors who hunted and foraged prior to farming was that they were food deprived and constantly on the verge of starvation but more recently this view has been challenged thanks to new evidence.

## The original affluent society

The 'original affluent society' was a phrase coined in 1966 by the anthropologist Marshall Sahlins,[2] who challenged the notion that our hunter-gatherer ancestors lived frugal and food/energy-deprived lives, always on the brink of starvation. Basing his ideas on the work of many anthropologists who studied surviving hunter-gatherer groups, such as the !Kung of southern Africa, Sahlins claimed that our ancestors enjoyed a wide and nutritionally diverse diet, and their dietary needs were met from abundant availability of fauna and flora. He also stated that such groups could satisfy their material requirements by working around 15 to 20 hours per week. Their lives may have been short (up to 55 years' lifespan) and often violent, with high infant mortality, but survivors of infancy were largely robust and healthy — findings that are confirmed by modern scientific paleopathology. This view suggests that such groups easily satisfied the first condition of all life — that of energy homeostasis (balance) whereby energy expenditure met energy income.

We have a wonderful window into the diet of ancient hunter-gatherers from around 750,000 years ago at the Gesher Benot Ya'aqov site in Israel, as described in a paper published in the journal *Science* in 2004.[3] The team led by Yoel Melamed found evidence of fire use and a wide variety of 55 plant species, sources of energy and nutrition, including nuts, fruit, seeds and root vegetables. There was evidence of both aquatic and terrestrial animal foods. This excellent study suggests that Shalin's hypothesis of the first affluent society might have been close to the mark.

## The diseases of civilisation

Then around 12,000 years ago and coinciding with the end of the last Ice Age, human behaviour changed, with the large-scale transition from a hunter-gatherer lifestyle to one of agriculture and settlement that allowed for an increasingly large population. The archaeological record shows us that this marked important changes in health, with average height reducing and the appearance or increase of the 'diseases of civilisation' – non-communicable diseases associated with lifestyle.

The diseases of civilisation include acne, obesity, diabetes, heart disease, cancer, early ageing and neurodegeneration. Essentially, they are diseases of increasingly high energy input and activate a key metabolic pathway, known to bioscientists as mTOR – and more popularly as the 'ice cream pathway' – that is, excess consumption of energy. This excess energy can be in the form of fat or sugars.

There is no doubt that the spread of industrial farming and food processing in the 20th century increased the incidence of these diseases, but it was the late 20th century that saw the concurrent explosion of refined carbohydrate and sugar consumption and the sudden increase in metabolic (energy dysregulation) conditions. This was when refined carbohydrates and sugars were increasingly added to our diets, and fats removed.

*Table 1: Numbers of studies published in a given year indexed in PubMed as an indicator of trends in research interest in sugar consumption and the four 'sugar sickness syndromes'*

| Year of publication | Sugar consumption | Obesity | Type 2 diabetes | Alzheimer's | ASD |
|---|---|---|---|---|---|
| 1970 | 321 | 784 | 2 | 11 | 78 |
| 1980 | 250 | 1348 | 7 | 110 | 111 |
| 1990 | 276 | 1944 | 1032 | 1361 | 188 |
| 2000 | 462 | 4640 | 2505 | 6062 | 368 |
| 2010 | 1122 | 16.600 | 7262 | 6896 | 1447 |
| 2020 | 2182 | 33,215 | 13,488 | 14,206 | 5776 |

## Cardiovascular disease – the driver of radical change in dietary recommendations

The American College of Cardiology has reported that the earliest documented case of coronary atherosclerosis (plaque build-up in the arteries that narrows the passage for blood flow and can cause a heart attack) was in an Egyptian princess who lived between 1580 and 1550 BC and that heart attack was more common in ancient times than previously thought.[4]

In more recent times, while narrowing of the arteries and angina were both known and discussed in 18th and 19th century Europe and America, we can quote Dalen and colleagues (2014) in saying that 'Heart disease was an uncommon cause of death in the US at the beginning of the 20th century. By mid-century it had become the commonest cause... due to an increase in the prevalence of coronary atherosclerosis...associated with an increase in smoking and dietary changes'.[5]

Americans were aware of this change but it was in 1955 when their President, Dwight Eisenhower, suffered a heart attack (myocardial infarction) while playing golf in Denver that something of a cardiovascular panic spread across the US. What was the cause and how could the problem be reversed?

We must remember that at this time the tobacco industry was in denial about the harmful effects of smoking and it was diet that was focused on as the likely cause.

High cholesterol levels were advanced as a major negative influence on heart health, and fats soon became health enemy number one. The good old American hamburger was blamed – Eisenhower had lunched on a hamburger before his heart attack. However, there was at that time already available sound science implicating high carbohydrate consumption as a major cause of metabolic dysregulation and weight gain.

## The fat versus sugar debate: Ancel Keys versus John Yudkin

Ancel Keys was the most famous American physiologist of the 20th century. He developed the K-rations that fed American soldiers during combat in WWII. He conducted important studies on starvation in men during that war, studies that have yielded profound information on human responses to starvation and from which lessons are still being learned.

Keys also conducted a famous investigation into diet that became known as the Seven Countries Study. This was the first study to examine systematically the relationship between diet and other lifestyle factors and rates of heart attack and stroke in contrasting populations. On the basis of the findings he reported, he claimed that cholesterol was a key factor in coronary heart disease.[6] In 1956, the American Heart Association accepted his findings and recommended that Americans reduce their consumption of butter, lard, eggs and beef to lower their risk of heart disease.

Other scientists criticised the findings of the Keys' study, but their voices went unheard. As we now know, Keys was selective in the data he reported, excluding countries that did not fit the model and ignoring the fact that the same data equally implicated sugar – countries eating higher amounts of fat were simultaneously eating more sugar.

Keys opposed the work of John Yudkin, a leading UK researcher into nutrition who focused on sugars as the major factor in causing heart disease, and wrote the recently republished book, *Pure, White and Deadly*.[7] Keys decisively won that battle, and his work became the yardstick for nutritional science. His views found their way into the famous Senate (McGovern) Committee's views on nutrition, and the bad-fat, good-sugar die was cast. This committee (known as the United States Senate Select Committee on Nutrition and Human Needs) met from 1968 to 1977. Although its dietary conclusions were not very radical, and John Yudkin testified to the committee, the members could not accept Yudkin's ideas because he opposed the dogma that fats were the major factor.

The food industry pounced on the 'bad fat' theory. Fats have a shorter shelf-life than refined carbohydrates and saturated fats (the ultimate villains) were more expensive as food products than either carbohydrates or unsaturated fats. Fats – especially saturated fats – were removed from foods and sugars added. The notion that fats caused heart disease soon transmuted into the notion that they also caused obesity and type 2 diabetes, which in turn morphed into a dogma. Since that time we have had an epidemic of obesity and diabetes and today heart disease remains the leading cause of death in the US despite a major decrease in smoking. In that time, has consumption of fats increased? Researchers Stephen & Sieber (1985) quoted a review of all published studies in the US that found 'fat intake has fallen steadily since the mid 1960s' and in their own review of 97 studies relating to the UK, fat represented 30% or less of dietary energy in the UK until the 1930, when it began to rise... reaching a plateau of 40% energy in the late 1950s with little change until the late 1970s when it began to fall.'[8]

If sugar consumption went up while fat consumption and smoking went down, coinciding with an explosion in obesity and related disorders, what are we logically to conclude?

### Hamburgers and heart disease: 2018 – a new perspective

Fast forward to March 2018 and this tragic story takes another twist. A group of scientists based in the Faculty of Sports Studies at the Masaryk University in the city of Brno, Czech Republic, published a historic study that not only overturned the work of Keys in the Seven Countries Study but also comprehensively demolished it with regard to heart disease.[9] The contribution that these scientists have made to the science of nutrition is extraordinary and should go down in the annals of medical science as one of the most important in the history of nutrition and energy metabolism; they have brilliantly and definitively settled the argument in favour of the bad-sugar hypothesis.

*A paper published in 2018 looking at data from 158 countries showed high-carbohydrate consumption to be the dietary factor most consistently linked with the risk of CVDs.*

They did not review information from a few selected countries as did Keys, but analysed nutritional and other factors potentially associated with the incidence of cardiovascular diseases (CVDs) globally from 158 countries, comparing the intake of 60 food items between 1993 and 2011, and their influence on obesity rates, health expenditure and life expectancy. Their conclusions were stunning and historic: they found that, regardless of the statistical method used, the results always showed very similar trends and identified high-carbohydrate consumption as the dietary factor most consistently associated with the risk of CVDs. Here at last we have the scientific truth after half a century!

## Yes, but do fats increase blood glucose concentration?

There is one last point to make about the fats versus sugars debate. One of the arguments against fats has been that increased circulating fats do cause insulin resistance (see page 99) and insulin resistance is a leading contributor to hyperinsulin-aemia and increased blood glucose concentrations. However, it should be noted that most of the fats that are released into the circulation come from our fat stores and that these directly result from consumed sugars that have been converted to fat and deposited in our adipose tissues. Furthermore, in recent decades consumption of fats has not risen significantly but consumption of refined carbohydrates and sugars has, dramatically.[10]

# The four sugar-enslavements of *Homo sapiens*

## The origins of the deadly human–sugar romance

Sugar from sugar cane originated in the Indian subcontinent and south east Asia in ancient times, where the plant was indigenous and was chewed for the pleasure of its sweetness, and where it was first domesticated. It was transported to the West and was known to the Greeks and the Romans as a medicine and luxury. The Venetian empire produced sugar for export to Europe in the near east, and in the 15th century the crop was being grown in the Canary Islands. In 1492, Christopher Columbus acquired cuttings from the Canary Islands and transported them to the island of Hispaniola (modern-day Haiti), where it was first planted in the New World. Sugar mills were soon created in Cuba and Jamaica, and later that century, under the colonial power of the Portuguese, the industry flourished in Brazil, which remains today one of the world's largest producers.

For the first time, refined sugar in industrial quantities could be relatively easily and cheaply produced for a newly wealthy market that could not get enough of this sweet stuff. Here was the beginning of what I call the four sugar-enslavements of our species, under which we continue to suffer:

1. The Atlantic Slave Trade and its legacy
2. Addiction to sugar
3. Obesity and the other sugar-sickness syndromes
4. Corruption of scientific intellectual capital.

## The first sugar-enslavement: The Atlantic Slave Trade

It was the demand for sugar that created the Atlantic triangular trading system and the Slave Trade, beginning in the early 16th century and lasting for almost three centuries. The early growers required cheap labour to cut, prepare and mill the sugar cane and this role was rapidly filled by African slaves from the western coastal regions of that continent. Sugar was transported from the Americas and Caribbean to Europe, where it was sold and exchanged for goods. From Europe, manufactured goods, such as textiles and arms, were transported to West Africa and bartered for slaves. The cycle was repeated at huge cost to life and liberty. Sugar was the economic commodity driving the wealth of European colonial powers – namely, the British, French, Dutch and Portuguese.

In Britain, the vast profits of the slave traders provided much of the capital that ultimately fostered the Industrial Revolution. It is thought that sugar alone accounted for one third of the European economy during these centuries. According to the scholar Henry Louis Gates Jr, the estimated number of slaves transported to North and South America was around 12 million. It is not unreasonable to state that the initial wealth of the British Empire was generated on the backs of many of those slaves.

On the 5th of July 1852, Frederick Douglas, an American abolitionist, writer, orator and escaped slave, delivered what has become the greatest abolitionist speech in American history: *What to the Slave is the Fourth of July?*. Included are these searing words:

> '... *Americans! Your republican politics are flagrantly inconsistent. The existence of slavery in this country brands your republicanism as a sham, your humanity as a base pretence, and your Christianity as a lie. It destroys your moral power abroad; it corrupts your politicians at home. It saps the foundation of religion; it makes your name a hissing, and a byword to a mocking earth. It is the antagonistic force in your government, the only thing that seriously endangers your Union. It fetters your progress; it is the enemy of improvement, the deadly foe of education; it fosters pride; it breeds insolence; it promotes vice; it shelters crime; it is a curse on the earth that supports it; and yet, you cling to it, as if it were the sheet anchor of all your hopes. Oh! Be warned! A horrible reptile is coiled in your nation's bosom; the venomous creature is nursing at the tender breast of your youthful republic; for the love of God, tear away, and fling from you the hideous monster, and let the weight of twenty million crush and destroy it forever!*'

Abolition came in the British Empire in 1807, though slaves in the British colonies were only freed in 1838 when the slave-owners (not the slaves) received compensation. In the US it came after the end of the Civil War, in 1865, but we are all now aware that the suffering did not end with 'freedom' and the legacy of this terrible exploitation is still playing out today.

# The second sugar-enslavement: Addiction to sugar

In November 2012, the *Daily Record*, a Scottish Newspaper, carried an article about a 51-year-old Scotsman, Andrew McSherry, who had undergone a quadruple heart bypass as a result of his addiction to a famous local drink, Irn Bru, which had such a high sugar content that his doctor concluded it had damaged his arteries. His cholesterol levels were sky high. Andrew had been addicted to the drink for 20 years, and consumed 8 litres daily, equivalent to 150 teaspoons of sugar over 24 hours, with an annual consumption of 272 kilos. He admitted that immediately after his operation he had purchased a bottle of the drink from the hospital trolley, but he had finally been persuaded to avoid it by his doctor, as a survival strategy.

Although Andrew McSherry represents an extreme example of modern humankind's quite recent enslavement to sugar, his addiction and health outcome are indicative of a global dependence on sugar that is increasing by the year, affecting not only the wealthy countries that developed its trade, but every country adopting a 'western' diet.

Global consumption of sugar in 2019-2020 amounted to 171.69 million metric tons. That figure is so huge as to be meaningless, but strikingly this consumption is projected to increase to about 178.84 million tons by 2023/2024. As the author of this report says: 'With the increase in world trade, better agricultural technology, among other reasons, sugar is cheaper and more widely available than ever.'[11] The US remains the biggest consumer on the globe at an estimated 126.4 grams per person per day, with Germany coming second at an estimated 102.9 grams per day. In both cases, the majority of this sugar is contained in processed foods such as cakes, pastries, sweets and fizzy drinks/sodas. Third is the Netherlands at 102.5 grams, fourth Ireland at 96.7 grams, fifth Australia at 95.6

grams and sixth the UK at 93.2 grams per person per day.

While saturated fats may continue to get most of the blame, there is general awareness that a high-sugar diet is bad not only for dental health, but for high blood pressure, heart disease and type 2 diabetes. Yet it seems we are unable to stop consuming sugar; we are *addicted*. But this addiction is costing us dear, rapidly destroying the physiological, psychological and cognitive health of our species, both before and after birth. As discussed throughout this book, sugar is a life-giving fuel, but excess sugar consumption is toxic, neurodegenerative, disease generating and potentially lethal.

## The third sugar-enslavement: Obesity and the other sugar sickness syndromes

For most of the history and prehistory of humans, the acquisition and consumption of the necessary energy resources to maintain all the functions of life, including reproduction of new generations, has been the major goal and influence on behaviour. Prior to the domestication of plants and animals, our hunter-gatherer ancestors appear usually to have been well provisioned (see page 14), except in the more weather-extreme regions of the world.

After the introduction of farming, food production rapidly increased, along with the population, but that dividend was subject to weather and pestilence, and was always vulnerable. Famines became a regular hazard. As civilisation developed, adequate food resources became more associated with the ruling strata in society, and classes evolved that could expropriate these at the expense of others.

Obesity, a condition of energy accumulation, is not new, but until the 20th century was associated almost exclusively with power and prosperity. Malnutrition was universal around the world, and hunger was still a major health concern in the USA as late as the 1960s. The initial impetus for the formation of the McGovern Committee in 1969, which became a major, if indirect, influence on the epidemic of obesity in America (see page 18), was not overconsumption of calories; it was quite the opposite – malnutrition. Diseases such as kwashiorkor (severe protein deficiency) and marasmus (calorie deficiency), which were common in underdeveloped countries, were present in the USA at that time. Only later did the Committee focus on overnutrition and, in 1977, issued a new set of guidelines.

At that time, the growth of heart disease had become a national obsession and fats were thought to be the major influence as described earlier (see page 17). This notion was supported by a powerful faction of the academic community, and thus began the war against fats and in favour of carbohydrates that coincided with the massive increase in worldwide adult and child obesity that continues to this day. Yes, fats do contribute to weight gain and obesity, but only under the control of insulin, the sugar hormone. Sugars are the initiating and key influence. This is very simply confirmed by the knowledge that fat consumption has not significantly increased from that period until now (see page 18). The issue of insulin, 'insulin resistance' and hyperinsulinaemia (chronically raised insulin levels) is one that we will come back to (see page 59) as it is an essential part of the puzzle.

Obesity is associated with an increased risk of heart disease, stroke, type 2 diabetes, dementia, cancer, osteoarthritis and depression. As I will explain in subsequent chapters, overconsumption of sugar is the upstream key to the development of all these conditions, but my chief focus in this book is on the neurodegenerative diseases, including Alzheimer's disease at the end of life and autism at its beginning.

## The fourth sugar-enslavement: Corruption of scientific intellectual capital

It is my view that sugar has corrupted and enslaved the intellectual capital of world academia for five decades. In the same way that the tobacco industry avoided scientific scrutiny for several decades by recruiting academics to support its claims that nicotine was not addictive, and that smoking was not unhealthy. Likewise the fossil fuel industry has been able to corrupt the environmental sciences in relation to their influence on global warming, and the sugar industry has been spectacularly successful in diverting the scientific community and the health establishment away from recognising the full toxicity of overconsumption of refined carbohydrates and sugars.

Intervention in scientific studies on sugar toxicity emerged in the 1960s, when the role of sugar in heart disease was first suggested. A body known as the Sugar Research Foundation (SRF) sponsored studies that diverted attention from sugar and focused on fats as the major influence. In 1965, the SRF sponsored a literature review published by the *New England Journal of Medicine*[12] that focused on fat and cholesterol as the key influences on heart disease, and the review downplayed the influence of sugars.[13] The role of the SRF was not disclosed.

This study represents one of the opening salvos in the future war between those who believed that fats were the major food that contributed to the increased obesity, type 2 diabetes and heart disease of the period, and those who believed that sugars were the culprit. Later, the sugar industry was directly involved in frustrating the work of Professor John Yudkin, the leading UK nutritionist who was one of the early pioneers in raising concerns about the negative health effects of sugars on human health, as discussed earlier (page 17); his work was viciously opposed, and his career thwarted. This intellectual corruption has continued into the 21st century.

In the 1970s, Robert Atkins emerged, a physician and cardiologist who had successfully treated overweight patients by advocating low carbohydrate and increased fat consumption to lose weight. This dietary approach became highly successful over two to three decades and Atkins wrote several books about it. During this time, I was a practising pharmacist and often discussed this issue with other health professionals. The response was universal – they invariably condemned him as a dangerous lunatic. If questioned further, they would mumble something like, 'Oh, too much protein is bad for you,' or 'Ketosis is dangerous'. It became clear to me that none of them had read Atkins, nor had they understood the role of benign ketosis in human energy metabolism, a survival strategy during famine or starvation and fasting.

*When health professionals described ketosis in the era of the Atkins Diet they confused it with dangerous ketoacidosis and contributed to the ongoing public confusion.*

As Madeline and Kelly Gibas reported, benign ketosis occurs during a high-fat/low-carbohydrate diet when glucose deficiency is overcome by conversion of fats to small fat molecules known as ketones that may supply the brain and other organs. It also occurs during famine and starvation to maintain fuel supply to the brain. It may be adopted to oppose some medical conditions, such as epilepsy, that are exacerbated by a high-carbohydrate/sugar diet. It is very different from ketoacidosis – a very dangerous condition that may occur in diabetes type 1 and late-stage diabetes type 2. When health professionals described ketosis in the Atkins era, they confused it with ketoacidosis, and contributed to the public confusion that continues to this day.[14]

Ketones are small fat molecules that the brain may use when glucose is in short supply. The health professionals who thought ketosis was dangerous were simply repeating the 'bad fat' dogma advanced in medical journals and research circles at the time. This was a period during which fats were being removed from foods and sugars added – and still the neurodegenerative diseases advanced. Supermarket shelves were packed with food labels proclaiming their 'low fat' health status, and still are. Something was intellectually wrong in the state of medical science.

In January 2017, a study was published in the *American Journal of Preventive Medicine*, by Daniel G Aaron and Michael B Seigel from Boston University, Massachusetts called 'Sponsorship of National Health Organisations by Two Major Soda Companies'.[15] The authors investigated soda company sponsorship of US health and medical organisations, and corporate lobbying expenditures connected with soda- or nutrition-related public health legislation from 2011 to 2015. The results were shocking: from 2011 to 2015, the Coca-Cola Company and PepsiCo sponsored 95 national health organisations, including those fighting obesity. They lobbied against 29 public health bills aimed at reducing soda consumption. They lobbied against public health intervention in 97% of cases.

*From 2011 to 2015 the Coca-Cola Company and PepsiCo sponsored 95 national health organisations, including those fighting obesity.*

If that seems bad, it gets worse. The sugar companies in Europe and the USA are subsidised to the tune of billions of pounds, euros and dollars. In 2004, Oxfam reported that the EU subsidised three major sugar companies $976 million. Britain's Tate and Lyle received €158 million out of that sum. In 2013, the US government subsidised the sugar companies $300 million.[16]

Sponsoring health and sporting organisations, and opposing health legislation, is expensive and, in the case of the sugar industry, it is the taxpayer who provides the funds. This is intellectual corruption on steroids. In essence, this means that the diseases that are crippling mankind physiologically, psychologically and cognitively are being subsidised by western governments, a crime of unimaginable dimensions, and one that threatens the cognitive demise of our species.

### Nutritional Lysenkoism: A western version

In the wake of Keys' influence and the McGovern Committee's conclusions (which were hijacked by the food/sugar lobby as we've seen), opponents of the bad-fat theory were marginalised, and their careers aborted. I regard this as a western version of 'Lysenkoism'.

Trofim Lysenko was a Soviet agronomist who opposed Mendelian genetics, and applied his ideas in agriculture, with disastrous results. However, he was supported by Joseph Stalin, and wielded great power and influence as Director of the Soviet Institute of Genetics. Those scientists who opposed him were dismissed, some were imprisoned, and some executed as 'enemies of the state'.

Here in the West, no scientists were imprisoned or executed for implicating sugars in metabolic diseases, but the negative effect of the bad-fat theory destroyed the careers of those who disagreed with it. In addition, the lives of those who consumed the processed foods and beverages that were created and marketed resulting from that hypothesis were blighted. Millions (now billions) of late-modern humans who were born around the middle of the 20th century, their children and their grandchildren, have paid the price in terms of obesity, type 2 diabetes, Alzheimer's disease and autism spectrum disorders – a global catastrophe that continues today.

Nutritional Lysenkoism is not dead. In his wonderful book, Metabolical,[17] Robert Lustig outlines contemporary attacks on scientists who oppose the bad-fat/good-sugar hypothesis. In each case, the attacks have come from dietitians who adhere to that hypothesis. In these cases, the detractors do not engage in a scientific discussion and offer their evidence; they simply attempt to destroy the careers of those they oppose.

## Lack of diversity in the citation of scientific evidence

Related to the suppression of research findings and their authors that don't fit the accepted rhetoric is the selective attention paid to findings published outside the western scientific establishment. I draw attention to this in the list of references for this book as it is notable that some really significant findings from non-western institutions have been completely overlooked.

For example, a study by Hamed and colleagues from King Saud University in Riyadh has very important findings to convey about the the excito-toxic effects of increased glutamate (see page 149) as a result of impaired glutamine synthetase,[18] but has been cited in other papers just twice since publication in 2018 – presumably because the work was done in Saudi Arabia. I talk about this paper in more detail in Chapter 8.

*The brilliant 2017 study from Annamalai University, Tamil Nadu, showing the anti-ammonia benefits of quercetin has secured only one citation in the PubMed library since publication.*

In Chapter 9 I include the brilliant study by Kanimozhi and colleagues at Annamalai Univerity in Tamil Nadu, India. This demonstrates the anti-ammonia benefits of quercetin through its enhancement of the expression of glutamine synthetase.[19] This historic study has secured only one citation in the PubMed library – a shocking indictment of western science.

Nowhere has this blindness to non-western research been clearer than in relation to honey. For reasons I explain in Chapter 9, western science has avoided looking at the possible benefits of honey, but in the non-western scientific world there was no such omerta, and from the early 2000s studies began to appear from outside the western canon showing that honey did have significant health potential. These studies were from China, Japan, Korea, India, Malaysia, the Middle East, Africa and South America.

In July 2012, a study was published in the *International Journal of Biological Sciences* by three researchers at the University of Science, Malaysia, which opened a new field of investigation into honey.[20] Entitled simply 'Honey – a novel antidiabetic agent', it presented conclusions that were potentially explosive, reversing half a century of nonsense emanating from western health institutions, professions and academia. In the decade since, the study has gained a miniscule number of citations in PubMed – 34, of which only six have been from the western cannon, that is approximately 3.5 per annum. If the study had been nonsense, there would have been a tsunami of citations pointing out its flaws, and essentially closing the door on future investigations into the benefits of honey. No such tsunami occurred; only silence. Silence is a powerful weapon in scientific disputes – if you are unable to refute findings that you do not like, the usual strategy is to ignore them and hope they will go away.

# Chapter 3

# Glutamine synthetase:
# The engine of cognition,
# communication and language

## Neurones, glia and microglia

You will almost certainly be familiar with neurones, the brain cells that transmit electrical information signals, and with synapses, the gaps between neurones bridged by neurotransmitters. You may be less familiar with glia and with microglia. Glia are cells that surround and supply neurones with energy, and microglia are specialised glial cells that function as the brain's immune cells.

Neurones in the brain are essentially the 'thinking' communication cells. Although they are widely known and discussed by the public, they constitute around only 50% of the brain. The other less well-publicised cells are the glia, a name that derives from Greek and simply means glue. They are also known as astrocytes or astroglia because they are star-shaped. They were first discovered by Rudolph Ludwig Carl Virchow, a 19th-century German physician and anatomist whose work was influenced by the Scottish pioneer in cell physiology, John Goodsir. These cells were historically thought to be structural and without an important function. We now know this is not only incorrect – it is nonsense. They are vital for all brain functioning and provide the neurones with water, energy, oxygen and nutrients. If the glia are not functional, the brain dies

It is glia that house the all-important enzyme glutamine synthetase that I have mentioned several times already. They also house the metabolic process called the glutamate/

glutamine (G/G) cycle that is critical to fuelling consciousness and cognition. This enzyme and cycle will appear repeatedly in this book as together they are the engine of human cognition, communication and language, and thereby the engine that fuelled, and fuels, the science, technology, poetry, literature, art and music of our species.

---

### Albert Einstein and glia

Albert Einstein died in 1955. Although some scientists entertained anatomical expectations that his autopsy would show that he had a larger brain than most, and that this might explain his remarkable scientific insights, his brain was not large; indeed, it was relatively small. At his autopsy in Princeton Hospital the pathologist, Thomas Harvey, retained and preserved his brain for future study.

With family permission, Harvey offered segments of Einstein's brain to interested scientists in the hope of finding a link to his genius. In 1985, Marion Diamond at the University of California received a portion for study. Her interest was in glia, and she had found that rats in favourable environmental conditions developed higher ratios of these to neurones. When she examined Einstein's brain compared to others, she found that his also had a higher ratio of glia to neurones.[1] At the time the role of glia as housing the G/G cycle was unknown, and the critical role of glia only emerged in the scientific literature in the early 2000s.

---

## Microglia

Microglia, which are specialised glia, are the resident immune cells (macrophages) of the human brain. They constitute around 10% of brain cells. They are also present throughout the nervous system. In the healthy brain, microglia are maintained in a state of low-level activity and become fully activated only during invasion or other pathological events. They migrate to areas of invasion or damage, and act as scavengers that absorb and digest accumulating plaques, such as amyloid and tau proteins that damage cells. They also prune dead cells and other materials that may interrupt neurotransmission in the brain. They are sensitive to any pathological damage to the brain and spinal column.

Essentially, they are the active housekeepers of the central nervous system and exert important neuroprotective functions. They attack invading infective organisms via the release of inflammatory signals and molecules that alert the brain and cause apoptosis (controlled cell death) in damaged cells, to protect healthy neural functions. If microglia are over-activated, as they appear to be in energy-dysregulated diseases, they mutate from neuroprotective to neurodegenerative via a tide of inflammatory and oxidative inflicted damage, as will be shown in later chapters.

## The pumping cycle that fuels human consciousness

Consciousness is a big deal. We know this because, if we lose it, we are in trouble. There are occasions when we agree to suspend it, such as during surgery when we wish to avoid pain and we are anaesthetised by health professionals under strictly controlled conditions. What consciousness is has been debated for thousands of years and the debate continues to this day, but we know approximately what it is by losing it, and then recovering.

It seems to exist in the brain – we may describe it as 'the mind' – and it has something to do with being aware both of ourselves and of the environment in which we exist. We are confident that we have it, that some other advanced living creatures, such as other primates, may have it but that others, such as bacteria, probably do not. We also know it is expensive in terms of energy, because if we lose the energy supply to the brain, such as during a fall in blood glucose concentration (hypoglycaemia), we rapidly lose consciousness and, if the energy supply is not quickly replenished, a coma may result, with death not far distant.

A sufficient supply of energy for the brain is therefore our highest priority. The brain, however, has no internal fuel store and consequently relies exclusively on the efficient functioning of a fuel pump to maintain its energy supply. This pumping system is an exquisite enzyme-driven cycling mechanism that, for every turn of its cycle, pumps a glucose molecule into the brain. This is the glutamate/glutamine (G/G) cycle enabled by the enzyme glutamine synthetase.[6]

Essentially the G/G cycle is a four-step circular process, analogous to a four-stroke cycle in a mechanical engine. (A four-stroke cycle consists of four distinct strokes: intake, compression, power and exhaust). This should not be surprising because the human brain consumes fuel, creates heat and performs work and therefore itself functions as an intellectual combustion engine.

The steps in the G/G cycle are:

1. When a neurone is energy deficient it sends glutamate as a hunger signal to the glia that supplies it.
2. In the glia, toxic glutamate is immediately converted to beneficial glutamine by the enzyme glutamine synthetase.
3. Glutamine is sent from the glia to the neurone.
4. Glutamine is converted back to glutamate, completing the cycle, and the glutamate is safely stored in secure bubble-like 'vesicles' until required for the next cycle.

*Figure 2: The glutamate-glutamine cycle*

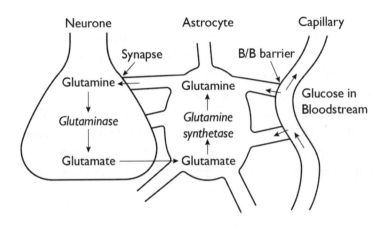

1. When neurones are low on energy, they release glutamate from vesicles and send it to astrocytes (glia).
2. Neurotoxic glutamate is the brain's hunger signal, and the enzyme glutamine synthetase converts it to benign glutamine.
3. Each turn of this cycle pumps a glucose molecule into the astrocyte from the bloodstream.
4. Glucose is split (glycolysis) into two lactate molecules, and these are sent to the neurone to provide energy (each lactate provides half the energy of glucose).
5. The glutamine is sent to neurones and reconverted to glutamate via the enzyme glutaminase.
6. The toxic glutamate is stored in vesicles to protect the neurone, and is released to restart the cycle, when required.

In more detail, the cycle begins with glutamate, which functions in a similar way to the spark plug in an internal combustion engine. As soon as excitotoxic glutamate enters the glial cell it must be converted to benign glutamine, to prevent toxicity. Glutamine synthetase performs this vital function. This conversion requires energy, and a glucose molecule is pumped into the glial cell with each turn of the cycle. A very small amount of the energy from the glucose is used to fuel the conversion of glutamate to glutamine, and most of the energy is sent to the neurone, to perform its work. Additionally, glutamine carries a second nitrogen atom compared to glutamate, which has only one, and this prevents the accumulation of ammonia, which is also highly toxic to brain cells (see below). Glutamate itself is highly toxic (excitotoxic) and, when converted from glutamine in neurones, is stored in special vesicles to protect the cell from damage.

Glutamine synthetase is consequently essential to life, and loss or absence of this enzyme is incompatible with life. Impairment is incompatible with healthy cognition, communication and language. This enzyme is also profoundly neuroprotective by virtue of its control of glutamate and ammonia levels in the brain, two of the most toxic molecules known in human energy regulation. It is also essential for healthy development of the nervous system. A recent study (March 2022) published in the *International Journal of Molecular Sciences* focused on the critical role of the glutamatergic system in neurodevelopment,[2] including synaptogenesis, synaptic plasticity, axon and dendrite formation and cellular migration, essential to the structure and function of the new brain. The authors looked at how this related to autism spectrum disorders.

## The benefit of cycles

Nature loves cycles. Without cycles there would be no life on earth. The Earth cycles around the sun, at the optimum distance that favours life in the 'Goldilocks Zone', neither too hot, nor too cold. There are astronomical cycles, solar and lunar cycles, other planetary cycles, climate cycles, geological cycles, light/ dark cycles, seasonal cycles and, in life, biological cycles. Some astrophysicists believe that the universe cycles through expansion, contraction and expansion again. Humans articulate circadian cycles, sleep/wake cycles, feeding/fasting cycles, menstrual cycles, life/death cycles. In economic and social life, humans index agricultural cycles, mathematical cycles, social cycles, monetary cycles… the list is very long.

If nature, biology and humans all share a love of cycles, it may be asked why do cycles occur so frequently in living systems?

## *Regulation*

The beauty of a cycle in any realm is that it offers the possibility of control. In any system, each turn of a cycle brings the various elements back to where they began, and each new rotation prevents an uncontrolled forward motion.

Life in a violent, unstable and often hostile environment is fragile, exceedingly fragile. All survival depends on maintenance of some level of equilibrium within very strictly controlled parameters of temperature, hydration, acidity and energy income/expenditure. For any living organism, including humans, any rapid alteration in these conditions requires a regulatory response to re-establish the optimal conditions required for survival. Human and other life forms have evolved highly sophisticated systems to regulate these factors in so far as is feasible for survival. Living or biological cycles function to solve problems, the most important of which is regulation of energy income. Energy is intangible, difficult to pin down, a force of work or heat or light, and always highly dangerous. Any system, mechanical or biological, that uses energy must regulate its income and output such that it is controlled.

During the Industrial Revolution, when humans harnessed huge quantities of energy to drive engines and machines, or create armaments, violent explosions were a regular hazard. They still occur. Life systems have evolved multiple mechanisms to take in, store and control energy in such a way as to fund generation, growth, reproduction and survival, and to protect against any damaging consequences. For example, the human immune system generates heat energy in the form of inflammation to attack invading organisms, but the resulting fever may be lethal to the human if it rises too high.

The human brain is a finely tuned internal combustion engine, and like any gasoline/petrol engine, must be sparked or fired to ignite the motion of the cylinders. The sparking mechanism in the brain is the highly toxic amino acid glutamate, and this ignites the enzyme cycle that pumps glucose into the brain. Each ignition must be matched by balanced inhibition. Excess glucose suppresses the inhibitory mechanism, the brain is thereby deprived of glucose/energy and the excitotoxic incendiary principle, glutamate, builds up, causing catastrophic damage to neurones and their synapses, resulting in cell death and brain shrinkage.

## Glutamate toxicity

Glutamate is the most abundant neurotransmitter in the human brain and nervous system. It is also profoundly excitatory, and is the major stimulatory amino acid in 90% of synapses. Its excitatory function is essential for a healthily functioning brain, but if high levels accumulate in the brain, it becomes highly toxic and is a major causal influence in, and marker of, neurodegenerative decline. High levels of glutamate have been identified in obesity,[3] diabetes type 2,[4] Alzheimer's disease[5] and autism spectrum disorders.[6] As we have seen, the enzyme glutamine synthetase converts toxic glutamate to benign glutamine to make it safe; glutamine deficiency is an emerging signal of cognitive decline in modern excess sugar-consuming humans.

## Glutamine deficiency

Glutamine is regarded as a 'non-essential' amino acid, meaning that humans can synthesise it and it is therefore not a required dietary constituent. However, the scientific literature describes it as *conditionally essential*; this refers to its un/availability during pathological conditions that prevent its synthesis in sufficient quantity to meet survival requirements. If such a condition became universal in modern humans, glutamine consumption would become increasingly essential. As I show in this book, excessive sugar consumption is suppressing the enzyme glutamine synthetase, essential for cycling glutamate back to glutamine and thereby resulting in reduced production of glutamine.

Interestingly, severe Covid-19 infection has been identified as a condition associated with glutamine deficiency.[7] Covid-19, like many viral infections, is a condition that causes what is known as 'viral hyperglycaemia'. Hyperglycaemia (overly high blood glucose) is the key oxidative mechanism that impairs glutamine synthetase, in the brain and body, as you will see in the next chapter, and glutamine synthetase is the only enzyme that converts glutamate to glutamine. To add to the vicious cycle, glutamine is also required to synthesise glutathione, the human body's most important antioxidant to counter oxidative stress.

---

**Stanley Lloyd Miller and glutamate**

In the chemistry laboratory of my school in the late 1950s, I recall the excitement generated when our science teacher told us about the work of Stanley Lloyd Miller and his experiments. Stanley Lloyd Miller is a hero in the life sciences and of this book, due to his idea of mimicking the conditions on Earth that gave rise to living entities from non-living chemicals. Miller was born in Oakland, California, in 1930. He attended Oakland High School where he was known by his peers as a 'chem whiz', and continued his studies at the University of California at Berkeley. He was intrigued by the mystery of how living (organic) matter spontaneously morphed from non-living chemicals in the so-called 'primordial soup'. He set out to see if he could demonstrate how this might have occurred.

Life is built from proteins that serve as the building blocks and the enzymes that drive all the machinery required for life to survive and function. Proteins are large and complex molecules but are composed of quite simple smaller molecules known as amino acids, found in all life forms. These consist of carbon skeletons with hydrogen, oxygen and nitrogen attached. ('Amino' refers to nitrogen atoms – each amino acid incorporates two nitrogen atoms.) There are around 20 amino acids humans need to make their proteins. How did the nitrogen get into these molecules? Miller questioned. In 1953, he sought to mimic the conditions of primitive Earth.[8] He fired steam into a mixture of methane, ammonia and oxygen, and applied an electrical charge into the vessel, perhaps mimicking a volcanic water-rich eruption and ancient electrical lightning storm. After a few days he found a few basic amino acids in the vessel, thereby conducting one of the most legendary experiments in the history of attempts to discover the origins of life. Miller had transformed the study of the generation of life for the first time in scientific history into a genuine field of research, now known as prebiotic chemistry.

In 2007 his original samples were reanalysed using modern, more sophisticated apparatus, and a significant number of additional amino acids were found to be present, including glutamate. We know that the glutamine synthetase gene is one of the oldest existing genes in the evolution of life (from 3.8 billion years ago),[9] so we may not be surprised to discover that glutamate is of similar age and, as the most common

neurotransmitter in humans, was present at the very birth of
neural sentience in all living organisms.

## Ammonia

When you use your household products you may be surprised
to learn that the active ingredient, ammonia, plays important
and essential roles in your own physiology, and that it may
also contribute to ill health in both body and brain if not
effectively regulated. Indeed, this compound is emerging as a
causative agent in cognitive decline that is associated with excess
consumption of refined carbohydrates and sugars.

Ammonia is a compound comprising one atom of nitrogen and
three of hydrogen ($NH_3$). It is a colourless gas and is widespread
in nature. It is toxic and dangerous and, if used as a cleaning
agent, must be handled with care. Nitrogen is essential to life,
since this atom is required as the critical structural element in all
amino acids that form proteins; proteins form the building blocks
and working machinery that drive all living systems. Ammonia
occurs naturally in the body, largely because of the breakdown
of amino acids, a process that releases free nitrogen, which is
converted to ammonia. In high concentrations, ammonia is toxic,
and it is eliminated from the body via the liver through a series
of reactions known as the urea cycle (another biological cycle!).
If liver function is impaired, ammonia concentration becomes
elevated in the blood, resulting in damage to the brain.

*Nitrogen is essential to build proteins but when the
body breaks these down, toxic ammonia results. We
need glutamine synthetase to clear ammonia from
the brain and the urea cycle to clear it from the body.*

The brain has a highly sophisticated system for controlling ammonia within safe limits – a system that depends on our friend, the enzyme glutamine synthetase and its conversion of glutamate to glutamine – adding nitrogen to glutamate with each turn of the G/G cycle. This critical cycle, as we have seen, prevents the accumulation of nitrogen and therefore of ammonia in the brain.

The hypothesis that ammonia might have a role in cognitive decline and Alzheimer's disease emerged in the early 1990s. Nikolaus Seiler at the Laboratory of Nutritional Oncology in Strasbourg, France, raised the alarm in 1993 in a paper published in the journal *Neurochemical Research*.[10] He found that elevated ammonia causes biochemical and cellular dysfunction in the brain, along with decreased energy metabolism and impaired neurotransmission, and increased glutamate neurotoxicity. Meanwhile, there is evidence to suggest that excess ammonia is a feature of obesity,[11] type 2 diabetes type 2,[12] Alzheimer's disease[13] and autism spectrum disorders.[14]

## The consequences of over and under supply of energy

During starvation, when glucose supply is limited or unavailable, the brain is given priority over other tissues so that survival may be possible. In the first phase, glucose is made from degraded proteins (mainly taken from muscle) in the liver, but that has only limited potential because most proteins are essential to life. After a few hours to a few days depending on the person's dependence on glucose, this process stops and fats are then broken down to form small molecules called ketones that the brain can use as fuel, as a strategy for survival. When fats are exhausted, proteins are again degraded, and this process indicates that the end is close.

The problem for most modern humans is not lack of brain fuel; rather it is excess fuel consumption. Throughout our history as a species, we have been subject to regular episodes of famine and starvation, but rarely to overabundance of foods, and certainly never to excess sugar. The human brain has therefore evolved no mechanisms to deal efficiently with this energy surplus. If the G/G fuel pump is overloaded it simply cuts out, and therein lies the origin of the modern crisis in cognition, communication and language. The human brain's fuel pump is suppressed, not acutely but chronically.

What are the consequences of suppressing the brain's fuel pump? In 2016 a study of (very rare) congenital glutamine synthetase deficiency[15] showed that this was associated with severe epileptic encephalopathy (a hallmark of autism), glutamine deficiency (a hallmark of excess sugar consumption) and chronically increased ammonia (a hallmark of all refined sugar-related conditions – obesity, diabetes type 2 and Alzheimer's disease). Clearly congenital deficiency of this vital enzyme is more potent than that induced by diet, but the indications are significant.

*Over-supply of energy is a new challenge for humans. Evolutionarily under-supply has been our problem.*

So how does diet suppress glutamine synthetase? As the next chapter will show you, this can result from oxidative stress caused by hyperglycaemia and from insulin resistance – a potential double-whammy for the brain.

## To summarise...

Before we look at the problems our 21st century diet is causing for glutamine synthetase in Chapter 4, it is useful to conclude this chapter with a reminder of this enzyme's essential functions. These are:

- controlling the use of nitrogen inside cells so that toxic ammonia and excitotoxic glutamate do not overwhelm our cells and we have enough glutamine to build proteins.
- regulating energy balance (homeostasis).

Given the dire consequences of not controlling nitrogen/ ammonia levels and not balancing energy supply with demand, we should clearly be doing all we can to support the optimal functioning of glutamine synthetase.

# Chapter 4

# Oxidising glutamine synthetase, the enzyme of human cognition

As we saw in Chapter 1, the human brain is very hungry and burns fuel at a very high rate. It also runs at a relatively high temperature (40°C and beyond),[1] making it particularly vulnerable to oxidative stress (damage), as described later in this chapter.

Humans acquire information via their systems of sensory perception of which there are five as you know: sight, smell, touch, taste and hearing. The sense organs collect environmental information via stimuli that are coupled with energy and integrated and encoded. Glutamine synthetase, the enzyme of cognition, is the engine of sense perception which couples and binds sensory information with the energy required for transduction into the nervous system and brain.

The role of information gathering (perception) is fundamentally driven by the glutamate/glutamine (G/G) cycle in both the brain and the peripheral nervous system, as described in Chapter 3. This was established by a team from the Department of Neuroscience at the University of Madrid in 2018.[2] They discovered that cognitive environmental information is integrated via information from the periphery via sensory neurones, which are key players in transduction and transmission of sensory information to higher centres, and that these neurones are tightly enclosed by glia that have glutamate receptors.

*Information gathering is fundamentally driven by the glutamate/glutamine cycle throughout the nervous system.*

This was beautifully demonstrated in 2017 by Erika Palmieri and colleagues of Bari University, Italy, in an international study published in the journal *Antioxidants & Redox Signaling*.[3] In this ground-breaking paper the authors showed for the first time a metabolic mechanism that mediates microglial response to a pro-inflammatory stimulus – that is, it implicates glutamine synthetase activity as a master modulator of immune cell function and shows that oxidative stress is the pro-inflammatory stimulant. This study, which in my view is worthy of a Nobel Prize, showed that microglia (the brain's immune cells) function as Ground Zero in each of the metabolic (energy dysregulation) diseases that are currently engulfing humanity, and that oxidative inflammatory degradation of glutamine synthetase, the enzyme of cognition, is the upstream mechanism defining all these diseases. The many negative pathways that drug manufacturers modify in the attempt to treat these conditions are all downstream from there.

## Oxidation

If you like avocados, you will know that they are nutrient dense and a very healthy food. They are rich in vitamins and minerals, include healthy fats, are high in dietary fibre and a variety of other health-giving nutrients, and have a low glycaemic index (they do not give rise to high blood sugar levels when eaten). However, you will also know that they are slow to ripen, and when they do so are edible for only a short time before rapidly turning brown and inedible. The browning is due to oxidation and is characteristic of other types of fruit such as apples and pears after peeling and exposure to oxygen in the air and light.

Oxidation is a form of combustion, when a fuel unites with oxygen. It can be explosive, such as in a bomb, or lower level such as in consumption of fuel in a vehicle, or, lower still, as in a burning candle. Although we think of combustion as a heat-producing reaction, in biological systems the heat produced is usually controlled. When a fresh avocado oxidises in air, some heat will be released, although at a level that is undetectable. All living beings use oxidation to release stored energy, and have numerous antioxidant systems that protect against the resulting oxidative damage.

The most dangerous activity in any cell is this controlled oxidation of fuel to release stored energy and thereby enable the cell to function. The higher the rate of consumption of fuel, the shorter is the lifespan. This applies to cells, organs, tissues and organisms, and seems to be a general rule across all living systems. Insects burn fuel at colossal rates and live very short lives. Elephants and whales burn fuel very slowly and have exceptionally long lives.

*Oxidation is essential to life but inevitable oxidative damage leads to ageing and death.*

Life cannot function and survive without oxidation. However, oxygen is also hostile to life. The life potential of any living organism is the result of the balance between the release of energy via oxidation and the efficiency of control of oxidative damage. All the energy-dysregulation diseases I examine in this book cause, and are caused by, oxidation, as evidence shows in obesity,[4] diabetes type 2,[4] Alzheimer's disease[5] and autism spectrum disorders.[6]

**Can information be oxidised?**

If cognition is information, and information is material (that is, a physical 'thing' as in 'the material world') cognitive information is subject to oxidation, as is all material. Every known material element, *including oxygen* is subject to oxidation. If information is material and affords mass, it is oxidisable.

On 4 March 2022, Dr Melvin Vopson of Southampton University, UK, published a revolutionary study in the journal *AIP Advances* that indicated information has mass and that all elementary particles, the universe's smallest building blocks, store information about themselves, similar to the way in which humans store information in DNA. This experiment, if confirmed, creates a new form of matter, in addition to solid, liquid, gas and plasma – information.[7]

We already know that energy and information are inseparable – if our smartphones run out of energy, the flow of information from or to the device ceases. Smartphones save lives in emergency situations and ensuring the necessary energy supply is critical to that function. Information is energy-expensive. Information technology data centres consume vast amounts of energy and generate heat. Cooling is energetically and economically costly. During a recent European heatwave, data centres were unable to cool down the heat generated, and services were halted. Information flow was suspended. As we may discover, this is not unlike the refined-sugar-generated overheating of the human brain that inhibits cognition.

## Inflammation

Every human is familiar with inflammation. From childhood we all know inflammation as the process that results from a cut or lesion – it hurts, swells, is highly sensitive to any touch or contact, and is usually hot and red. It is the reaction to any damaged tissue and performs two major functions – to attack and eliminate any invading organism or irritant, and to initiate recovery. The swelling results from immune cells that are deposited into the damaged tissue from the blood, increasing discomfort and pain. The **pain** is a protective mechanism to stop us using the tissue, and therefore to allow recovery to advance. (Professional athletes who are injured are often treated with pain-killers and anti-inflammatory medications to allow them to perform, but that is a dangerous strategy as the recovery will be incomplete, and the injury may be compounded.) The **heat** is antimicrobial – many invasive organisms cannot function above normal body temperature. Inflammation is a protective mechanism.

However, inflammation may be unhealthy in conditions where it does not resolve and/or is over-activated, including allergies and autoimmune diseases, such as arthritis. A variety of degenerative diseases also cause, and are caused by, excess inflammation, including atherosclerosis, heart disease, obesity,[8] type 2 diabetes,[9] Alzheimer's disease[10] and autism spectrum disorders.[11]

*Over-activation of microglia, the brain's immune cells, leads to inflammation and has been linked to neurodegeneration.*

Remember too that microglia are the cells in the brain that perform the key functions of the immune system, the equivalent of macrophages elsewhere in the body (see page 34). They attack invading infective organisms via the release of inflammatory signals and molecules that alert the brain and cause apoptosis (controlled cell death) of damaged cells, to protect healthy neural function. If microglia are over-activated, they mutate from neuro-protective to neurodegenerative via a tide of inflammatory and oxidative inflicted damage. There is evidence of microglial over-activation in each of the sugar sickness syndromes: obesity,[12] type 2 diabetes (diabetic retinopathy[13]), Alzheimer's disease[14] and autism spectrum disorders.[15]

## Losing touch with the environment – how our sensory abilities are being compromised, exemplified by vision

The role of information gathering (perception) is fundamentally driven by the G/G cycle providing energy for the nervous system, as we have seen (see page 47), in both the brain and the peripheral nervous system. This was established by a team from the Department of Neuroscience at the University of Madrid in 2018.[16] They discovered that cognitive environmental information is integrated via information from the periphery via sensory neurones, which are key players in transduction and transmission of sensory information to higher centres, and that these neurones are tightly enclosed by glia that have glutamate receptors – that means they use glutamate as a neurotransmitter. This sensory transduction of environmental information requires high energy, and glutamine synthetase is the enzyme that binds this information with the required energy for integration and encoding.

*Dysregulation of the enzyme glutamine synthetase is separating us from the environment as each of our senses is compromised.*

Vision provides a model for each of the other sensory pathways – hearing, smell, taste and touch – although the mechanical apparatus in each differs. The refined-sugar-driven loss of integrity and function of glutamine synthetase in the previous half century is the primary mechanism that is separating humans from the environment that nurtures them. Vision is not only the most acutely sugar-compromised sensory information pathway, but impaired vision is also the signal of sugar-impaired cognition in each of the metabolic diseases addressed in this book.

## Vision and the need for energy

Visual perception is the sensory ability to interpret the surrounding environment via light that is reflected by objects in that environment. Light enters the eye through the cornea, and is focused by the lens onto the retina, the light-sensitive membrane at the back of the eye, which transmutes the photons into electrical neuronal signalling. Retinal signals are transmitted via the optic nerve to the visual cortex in the brain. This sensory transduction of environmental information requires very high energy, and glutamine synthetase is the enzyme that binds this information with the required energy for integration and encoding. Vision information provides a model of how energetically costly information acquisition is, and how sensitive it is to any small decrease in energy provision.

Michael Denton of Otago University, New Zealand, has described the eye photoreception cell as the highest known consumer of energy compared to all other tissues.[17] He noted that the photoreceptor generated an electrical response to a single photon, a process that required vast quantities of energy. On a cell-for-cell basis, the human retina consumes three times the energy of the brain's cerebral cortex. Given this high demand, vision is the sensory perception system that is most sensitive to sugar-driven energy deficiency caused by oxidation of glutamine synthetase. It thereby provides a model both for the emergence of cognition 500 million years ago, and for its catastrophic decline in the last half-century.

## Vision and the ignition of cognition: The light switch

The eye and the brain are intimately linked together in the history of evolution. Indeed, it seems that they are so intimately related that without vision as the catalytic influence, cognition might not have developed as it did. Both of these vital evolutionary gains is today in decline, and that process is directly coupled with loss of energy in each system, due to excess circulating glucose suppressing the fuel pump that provides the energy that each function requires.

Complex eyes first appeared around 500 million years ago in the period known as the Cambrian. Prior to that time, small single-cell organisms in the Precambrian seas had developed primitive eyes, which were simply light-sensitive spots on their external membranes.

During the following period there occurred a colossal 'Cambrian Explosion' during which a rapid increase in bio-diversity occurred, when almost all the ancestors of animal species existing today appeared over a short period of time – around 25 million years, a mere blink of the evolutionary 'eye'. This sudden exponential diversification of complexity and form puzzled evolutionary biologists (including Charles Darwin) for a long time. However, Andrew Parker has solved the problem with his famous 'Light Switch Theory'.[18] He showed that the appearance of eyes sparked an evolutionary arms race, in which vision gave advantages to predators, and prey had to catch up or perish. Teeth and jaws emerged to aid predation, and internal bones and external hard parts and shells appeared to protect potential prey.

If we may say vision is the midwife of cognition, we may

also say that the eye is mother to the brain. The more acute the vision, the more complex is the diversification of form, and the more advanced is the primitive embryonic brain and cognition. Vision and cognition are evolutionary siblings, with vision as the slightly elder.

*Vision is the mother of cognition – our two most important evolutionary gains that are both now being compromised by a high-sugar diet.*

After advancing for half a billion years, and in our own species from around 200,000 years ago, both of these two evolutionary gains of function, vision and cognition, are now in retreat in Homo sapiens, and that regression is particularly clear in autism spectrum disorders, in which they are both attacked during neurodevelopment in the womb. The paediatric neurologist Professor Rubin Jure reported in 2019 that he had found autism was 30 times more prevalent in blind compared with sighted people, and that up to 50% of autistic children had visual deficits.[19] He also confirmed that this relationship was independent of intellectual ability, showing that cognition alone could not explain the connection.

Vision and cognition are two of our most important evolutionary gains. Both are facilitated and advanced by the enzyme glutamine synthetase. Both are attacked and compromised by excess glucose in the human circulation, as we know from the high risk of retinal damage in diabetes. If our hunter-gatherer ancestors had found a way to concentrate and refine plant sugars for consumption in our prehistory, they might have halted the visual and cognitive advances that have characterised our species until recently. We should be grateful that they did not, but hopefully we may learn from that period of low-sugar income before it is too late.

## *Light energy: Generating vision and cognition*

Energy and cognition are inseparable. Vision and cognition are inseparable. Light energy from the sun provides the fuel for all life forms in the form of sugars that are created from carbon dioxide and water via photosynthesis.[20] Light energy therefore performs the two critical functions that created the human brain and human cognition: the first was to provide the photosynthetic energy that fuelled all life forms, before and after the birth of vision; the second was to drive the formation of vision by activating light-sensitive membranes in the multitude of small, simple single-cell organisms that populated the seas some 500 million years ago. In other words, photosynthesis provided the energy that generated life, and photo-radiation stimulated light sensitivity in advance of vision.

## *Dimming the light switch: Oxidising vision and cognition*

Oxidation of sugars in living cells – sugars that are produced by photosynthesis – is the fundamental mechanism that releases the energy of life, as we have seen. However, excess consumption of refined sugars paradoxically drives oxidation of cellular machinery, and oxidative stress is the driving mechanism of the metabolic (energy dysregulation) diseases. For an organism to invite light into its metabolic machinery to enable vision is also to open its tissues to the most potent oxidising influence on earth – photo-energy. This double oxidative insult – light and sugars – explains why the eye is the most time-sensitive organ to oxidative damage in humans. Diabetic retinopathy is the largest contributing influence on global human blindness. The National Eye Institute (NEI) of America found that the disease increased from 4 to almost 8 million in the years from 2000 to 2010, and that this is expected to reach 14.5 million by 2050.[21]

The notion that both vision and cognition are intimately

related, as indicated by Rubin Jure's findings in people with autism and visual problems, was recently confirmed by Wing Shan Yu and colleagues in the journal *Annals of New York Academy of Sciences*.[22] They showed that electrical stimulation of the cornea (the light-refracting outer layer of the eye) improved cognition, a global gain of function in sensory perceptive environmental information processing, beyond vision alone. The importance of this finding should not be underestimated.

It is now increasingly recognised that chronic energy deficiency in the eye and brain, caused by oxidative degradation of glutamine synthetase, is the most potent driving force of inflammation and heat-death (pyroptosis) of neurones.[23]

## Oxidising cognition, communication and language: The shared downstream pathways

We know that the biological machinery of sensory cognition and its transmission from cell to cell is subject to sugar-driven oxidation, as exemplified by vision. Excess glucose in the bloodstream inhibits information-derived cognition by oxidising glutamine synthetase in glia, thereby depriving the brain of energy – the energy it needs to fund transferral of information and the dynamism that drives cognition, communication and language. This event is the upstream and defining mechanism in all the sugar-sickness syndromes that degrade human cognition, communication and language.

Alzheimer's disease is a condition of impaired cognition, communication and language as I will discuss in detail in Chapter 7. In this condition, the brain, including the hippocampus, shrinks. Andres Lozano, a Professor of Neurosurgery in Toronto, Canada, led a study published in the *Journal of Alzheimer's Disease* that rocked the scientific community of Alzheimer's researchers by reversing that trend.[24] He applied deep brain stimulation to the fornix, an area of the brain that transfers information to the hippocampus and consolidates short- and long-term memory. Over the course of a year, one patient had an increase of 5% in the hippocampus and another 8%. These were astonishing results and support my contention that this condition is one that results from low brain energy metabolism that follows oxidative degradation of glutamine synthetase, the only enzyme that pumps glucose energy into the human brain.

*Neurodegenerative diseases result from low brain energy metabolism following oxidative degradation of glutamine synthetase.*

It is doubtful if our species can solve its current and future cognitive decline by creating and wearing brain energy implants that would deliver the energy required to replace that which is lost due to refined-sugar-induced loss of glutamine synthetase. However, we may cease to sweeten our food or, as Chapter 9 will show, replace refined sugars with honey. The bioflavonoids in honey will protect glutamine synthetase, just as occurs in the honeybee every time it sets off from the hive. However, the successful application of deep brain stimulation in this key sugar-sickness syndrome has confirmed that these excess-sugar-driven conditions are characterised by, and share, chronic brain energy deficiency:

- obesity[25]
- insulin resistance[26]
- Alzheimer's disease[27]
- autism spectrum disorders.[28]

Before looking at each of these conditions in turn, it is important to look further at the overall factors driving their increase.

Chapter 4

# Insulin resistance and hyperinsulinaemia

Insulin is the hormone that promotes glucose transport into cells, thereby controlling blood glucose levels. Insulin resistance is a global condition affecting up to 40% of adults worldwide. It is associated with the condition metabolic syndrome, which is a risk factor for obesity and type 2 diabetes, and is characterised by cell membranes showing reduced sensitivity to insulin in the bloodstream; as a result, insulin increasingly fail to influence cellular uptake of glucose and the pancreas, in a frantic effort to maintain blood sugar at a normal level, pumps out increasing amounts of insulin to overcome the problem. Hyperinsulinaemia is the result – chronic abnormally high circulating levels of insulin in the bloodstream while blood sugar levels remain apparently 'normal'.

Insulin resistance has been associated with obesity,[29] type 2 diabetes[30] and Alzheimer's disease[31] and maternal insulin resistance with autism.[32] Hyperinsulinaemia and insulin resistance are mutually causative, a vicious cycle that adds to the negative health outcomes.

*Chronically high levels of insulin in the bloodstream lead to the brain being starved of energy.*

Insulin resistance developed in our evolutionary history as a survival strategy when food and energy were deficient, and the brain activated resistance to insulin to ensure that it, the brain rather than the body, had first access to vital fuel supplies. If body tissues are unable to take a full share of available circulating glucose, more will be available for the brain to use. (This is known as 'energy partition'.) In modern times, excess energy consumption paradoxically deprives the brain of energy, mimicking energy paucity, and the resulting resistance simply adds to the pathology. The brain is starved of energy.

A study published in the *Journal of Clinical Investigation*,[33] in 2000 by researchers at Harvard Medical School, USA, looked into the relationship between obesity, insulin resistance and hyperinsulinaemia. They discovered that insulin resistance and hyperinsulinaemia, in addition to being caused by obesity, might also contribute to its development.

In Chapter 8 on autism spectrum disorders, we will look at the pioneering work of Michael Stern at Texas University.[34] He found a connection between foetal hyperinsulinaemia and autism. Gestational diabetes doubles the risk of autism incidence and Michael Stern cites evidence that, although insulin does not cross the placental barrier, high levels of maternal glucose would cross into the foetal circulation and activate the high-energy pathways that are associated with autism (see page 130).

### *Improving insulin sensitivity*

The Gila monster is a venomous lizard that lives in the south-west United States and north-west Mexico. It is a slow-moving creature, about 2 feet (60 cm) in length, and feeds on small mammals, frogs, insects, birds and bird and reptile eggs. It is not a threat to humans, but it does have a nasty bite and has been killed out of fear. It is now a protected species. The venom can have powerful (usually harmful) effects on animals, including humans, and scientists have learnt much from its components and how they exert their effects.

John Eng, a scientist at the Bronx Veterans Affairs Hospital, New York, USA, became interested in the Gila monster because its bite triggered inflammation in the pancreas. He isolated a protein that closely resembled a human protein known as glucagon-like peptide-1 (GLP-1). GLP-1 improves blood glucose control. However, the human version was not useful in diabetics because it had a very short-acting lifespan in human serum, and its benefits could not be utilised. With some molecular modification, Eng's protein from the Gila monster proved much more beneficial, because it had a longer-lasting action, and eventually was developed into a drug – Exendin – used to treat diabetes.

*Chronically high levels of blood sugar block the brain's fuel pump, leaving the brain starved of energy and telling us we need to consume more energy, which keeps our blood sugar high.*

Exendin and a group of similar medications are now routinely used in type 2 diabetes. There is scarcely an organ or tissue on which GLP-1 and its longer-life medications fail to exert beneficial effects.[35] In the brain they are neuroprotective. We know that in conditions of chronically high blood glucose concentration (hyperglycaemia), the brain's fuel pump is blocked, and this energy deficiency activates brain hunger and therefore appetite. These medications act to prevent too much glucose crossing the blood-brain barrier, thereby reducing the danger of excess glucose in the brain which would have devastating consequences. You might therefore expect them to cause increased brain hunger, and therefore appetite. However, we also know that these medications reduce appetite. How may this paradox be resolved?

GLP-1 and its medical offshoots improve brain insulin sensitivity, thereby increasing the efficiency of glucose metabolism in the brain.[36] This is one of the most significant influences in improving each of the major metabolic (energy dysregulation) diseases, including obesity. Refined carbohydrates and sugars suppress the human brain's fuel pump, the enzyme glutamine synthetase. The brain is deprived of energy and this activates the appetite hormones. The cycle repeats.

Improving brain insulin sensitivity upgrades glutamine

synthetase,[37] an effect that would improve appetite. In effect these drugs add an extra control mechanism that is also neuroprotective. If by doing so they improve brain energy metabolism, it would not be surprising if they demonstrated benefits in obesity, a condition that is also driven by reduced brain energy metabolism. This effect has been confirmed by Dr Lucy Checke at the University of Cambridge who found that obesity is associated in the brain with reduced volume and memory deficits, confirming the neuropathology of weight gain.[38]

*Improving sensitivity to insulin upgrades glutamine synthetase, which normalises our appetite and gets rid of cravings.*

In 2017, Mayo Clinic researchers showed that liraglutide, a GLP-1-type medication, does stimulate weight loss in a study published in the *Lancet Gastroenterology & Hepatology*.[39] The study showed that liraglutide administered for three months at a dose of 3 mg per day generated an average of 5.5 kilos' (12 lb) weight loss. The authors attributed the benefit to the effect of slowed stomach emptying characteristic of this drug. However, the real site of action may well have been in the brain, where hunger arises, and where uncontrolled blood glucose concentrations exert multiple neurodegenerative mechanisms.

Modern humans are chronically overloaded with blood glucose. Improved glucose metabolism in the brain, by restraining extra glucose from crossing the blood-brain barrier and simultaneously improving glucose efficiency, along with reducing toxic glutamate in the brain, would potentially offer benefits in cognitive and memory disorders. Not surprisingly a drug known as Gilatide, derived from exendin-4, has been selected for research into potential benefits in Alzheimer's disease.[35] This drug affects sugars and not fats. This does not mean that fats are not involved – they are, but via insulin action, and insulin is predominantly a sugar-controlling hormone. Furthermore, the mechanism of action of these Gila-derived medicines is in the brain, and the brain does not normally burn fats to release energy.

## Glycation: Advanced glycation end-products (AGEs), iron deficiency and hypoxia

If you have ever viewed a bartender rimming a cocktail glass with sugar, you may note that the glass is first dipped into a liquid such as lemon juice to capture the sugar. This renders the sugar sticky before it is applied to the glass rim so that it will add sweetness to the drink. Sugar crystals are 'dry', and sugar-stickiness requires the crystals to be liquified. In the human circulation, sugar is dissolved, and excess circulating sugar (glucose) causes all kinds of metabolic problems by sticking to proteins and fats – a process known as glycation. Advanced glycation end-products (AGEs) are proteins and lipids (fats) that have been 'glycated' by exposure to excess circulating glucose. They are associated with modern degenerative diseases, including type 2 diabetes, atherosclerosis and kidney disease. They are increasingly found as significant markers of neurodegeneration and consequent cognitive decline because sugar-induced oxidation of glutamine synthetase in brain glia sets off an inflammatory conflagration that heat-destroys neurones via pyroptosis (inflammatory cell death).

There is evidence that AGEs are a biomarker in obesity,[40] type 2 diabetes,[41] Alzheimer's disease[42] and autism spectrum disorders.[43]

### *Iron-deficiency anaemia*

Haemoglobin is the specialised protein in red blood cells that transports oxygen in the human body and delivers it into the cells, organs and tissues that require it to burn fuel (glucose or ketones) and release the energy they need to function and survive. When concentrations of blood glucose rise and remain high over an extended period of time, they stick to and damage circulating fats and proteins, including haemoglobin, which is highly vulnerable. The product of this sticking (glycation) in red blood cells is known as HbA1c – glycated haemoglobin. High blood glucose concentrations are usually transient, and levels may vary quickly, but HbA1c remains once formed and is consequently a sensitive measure of blood glucose levels over time; it has become the standard measure used by clinicians to diagnose type 2 diabetes.[44]

*Hyperglycaemia causes oxygen loss in the cells lining brain blood vessels triggering the body to produce more haemoglobin and deplete its iron stores.*

Iron-deficiency anaemia is a common concern in modern humans worldwide, affecting up to 1.5 billion people. This condition, if not resolved, is deeply damaging to health and may lead to death. Its most damaging effects are found in pregnant women and in children. Iron deficiency is profoundly related to diabetes, and it has been shown to negatively affect glucose regulation. Excess glucose (hyperglycaemia) causes hypoxia (oxygen loss) in the cells lining the blood vessels (endothelial cells) that supply the brain. The brain is thereby deprived of oxygen and the body is prompted to release factors that increase production of haemoglobin; this increased supply of haemoglobin can then increase oxygen supply by increasing the capacity to transport it. However, haemoglobin is dependent on iron for its formation, so reserve iron stores are plundered and diabetes thereby develops into an iron-deficiency disease. Iron deficiency in turn dysregulates glucose control, and the toxic cycle continues. There is evidence of this in obesity,[45] insulin resistance,[46] dementia[46] and autism spectrum disorders.[48]

## *Hypoxia (under-supply of oxygen)*

Two of the leading causes of brain ischaemia (lack of blood supply) are obesity and type 2 diabetes, major conditions associated with overconsumption of refined sugars. The brain is deprived of oxygen and glucose, and its ability to generate survival energy fails. This triggers an oxidative storm in the glia, glutamine synthetase is suppressed, and inflammation and destruction of neurones follow. Failure to convert glutamate to glutamine results in excess glutamate excitatory signalling, calcium overload occurs, and the area of the brain affected is severely damaged.[49] This is an acute version of the chronic impaired brain metabolism (energy dysregulation) that is driven by refined-sugar impairment of glutamine synthetase expressed in each of the sugar sickness syndromes. Hypoxia is associated with each of these conditions – obesity,[50] type 2 diabetes,[51] Alzheimer's disease[52] and autism spectrum disorders.[53]

## Water, energy and cognition: Vasopressin and oxytocin

Water is essential to life. The human adult body is composed of about 60% water by weight. A loss of as little as 2% is sufficient to cause mental confusion. The brain is the organ most vulnerable to any water deficit. Water fills and enables cells to function, regulates temperature, is required for digestion, lubricates joints, insulates internal organs, carries all nutrients to cells including oxygen and glucose, and flushes out toxins and waste materials. Dehydration is a life-threatening condition.

Water enters the human brain via two systems:

1.  When glucose is pumped into the brain by the energy pump, glutamine synthetase, water is also carried over via osmosis, to match the higher concentration in brain cells. This system balances the pressure inside and outside of the brain.

2.   The blood pressure in the tiny blood vessels that supply the brain is slightly higher than the inside (intracranial) pressure, and this ensures a highly controlled, steady flow of water, oxygen and multiple nutrients into the brain so that this organ is supplied with all it requires to function and survive.

The two systems are exquisitely counterbalanced to ensure optimal function. If too little water reaches the brain (hypoperfusion), the brain will lack both energy and oxygen, and brain cells will quickly die. Excess water entering the brain (hyperperfusion syndrome) is also highly dangerous, due to increased pressure.

In 2006 two researchers, Elizabeth Hammock and Larry Young at the Center for Behavioural Neuroscience at Emory University, Atlanta, Georgia, USA, published an important paper in the *International Journal of Molecular Science* that should have rocked the scientific community but did not do so.[54] They focused on two seemingly unrelated hormones, one that modulates hydration (vasopressin) and one that modulates reproduction (oxytocin), and showed that they act on two of the most vital intersecting survival pathways in humans – hydration and energy. The authors stated that these two hormones contributed to various social behaviours, including social recognition, communication, parental care, territorial aggression and social bonding, and that disruption of these central neurological pathways offered insight into autism. This was an outstanding contribution to our understanding of modern refined-sugar-driven water/energy stress and consequent negative influences on cognition.

In any metropolitan street it is noticeable that, contrary to 20th century observations of earlier generations, many people carry water bottles. This relatively new phenomenon is associated with widespread water stress, which in turn is directly influenced by energy stress. Indeed, health advisers frequently recommend that people ensure they are sufficiently hydrated. This connection was confirmed by a 2011 study published in *Diabetes Care*.[55] The authors reported that water intake was inversely and independently associated with the risk of developing hyperglycaemia. Diabetes and prediabetes (metabolic syndrome) are each associated with water loss and thirst.

> *Water intake is inversely and independently associated with the risk of developing hyperglycaemia – the majority of modern humans are chronically water-stressed.*

As we have seen, each of the modern neurodegenerative diseases is characterised by chronic reduced brain energy metabolism due to excess sugar suppressing the brain's glucose pump – the enzyme glutamine synthetase. Given the above, it seems likely that this energy deficit will be accompanied by reduced water flow into the brain.

In 2018 a study published in the journal *Acta Neurobiologiae Experimentalis* by a combined team of researchers from Norway, USA, Chile, Egypt and Italy[56] found that cerebral hypoperfusion, and insufficient blood flow (ischaemia) in the brain, occurred in many areas of the brain in patients diagnosed with autism spectrum disorders. They also discovered that in individuals diagnosed with autism, there was a direct relationship between the index of autism pathology and the cerebral dehydration – the more autistic the individual, the greater was the water deficit in the brain. The authors made some suggestions as to how this water deficit might be addressed, none of which was practical – it simply did not occur to them that the most common condition worldwide that causes dehydration and extreme thirst was excess glucose circulating in the blood (diabetes) – the kidneys work hard to expel the excess sugar, and this carries water out of the body via the urine. If the brain is deficient in water due to hypoperfusion, thirst is its most potent signal, indicating that the brain is not only lacking in water but also in energy.

## Water not on the brain: Vasopressin

Physical exercise, and hot temperatures, impose severe water-deficit stress on humans. Therefore, exercise physiology provides valuable insights into the negative effects of dehydration on the human system. In November 2018, MT Wittbrodt and M Millard from the Exercise Laboratory at the School of Biological Sciences, Georgia Institute of Technology, USA, published an important paper in the journal *Medicine and Science in Sports and Exercise.*[57] The authors found that the magnitude of dehydration was associated with the level of impairment in cognitive performance.

*Hyperglycaemia leads to dehydration as the body flushes out excess sugar. Dehydration leads to cognitive impairment and confusion.*

Vasopressin is a hormone that protects against water loss in the human body and brain. It is released from special cells in the hypothalamus into the pituitary gland and from there into the circulation. The hypothalamus senses the extracellular water level and reacts when this is low and the concentration of molecules in blood and lymph rises too high, a dangerous event. The brain is therefore the first organ in the body to react to dehydration and seeks to avoid acute water stress. Vasopressin increases the amount of water reabsorbed from the fluid passing through the kidneys, and thereby protects against the dangers of dehydration. It is also notable that vasopressin is a neuroprotective hormone.[58]

Diabetes is a condition in which excess glucose in blood plasma results in dehydration, due to the kidneys excreting excess glucose in urine with consequent water loss and dehydration. The cycle continues – dehydration of the brain causes cognitive impairments. A synthetic version of vasopressin is provided to patients whose anti-diabetic medication may not sufficiently protect against dehydration.

### Energy not in the brain: Oxytocin

In 1906, an English pharmacologist, Henry Hallett Dale, discovered a hormone that stimulated contractions of the uterus (womb); this was later named oxytocin. Over the following century our knowledge of the range of functions that this hormone was involved in expanded dramatically. We now know it has an important role at every stage of life: reproduction, birth, lactation, parental bonding, child play behaviour, social interaction, social recognition, affiliation, sexual behaviour, social trust and social defence including aggression.

A June 2009 study published in the journal *Progress in Neurobiology* focused on the vital role of oxytocin at different life stages. It referred to oxytocin as the 'great facilitator of life', which seems an apt description for a hormone that intervenes at all the most critical transitions in the human life cycle, from birth to death, as described by the authors.

Oxytocin is produced in the region of the brain called the hypothalamus that regulates hunger and thirst and is released into the circulation via the pituitary gland. Although it has widespread effects throughout the body, its levels in the brain are around 1000 times greater than in the body. We should not be surprised therefore to discover that this versatile hormone is also involved in memory and cognition, and that energy regulation is the major area of action. Since cognition and its impairments are linked to the breakdown of energy regulation in the brain, it would seem likely that this hormone would also impact the major energy diseases that result directly from energy dysregulation in the human brain, including obesity and type 2 diabetes.

*Oxytocin levels are 1000 times higher in the brain than the body and this hormone, dubbed 'the great facilitator', is associated with memory, cognition and communication.*

This is exactly what a study published in September 2018 found.[59]The authors showed that plasma oxytocin concentrations were lower in obese individuals with diabetes and that oxytocin had emerged as an attractive target for treating metabolic energy dysregulation in obesity and diabetes.

Each of these conditions results directly from poor glucose/ energy transfer from body to brain, resulting in chronic brain energy deprivation, increased blood glucose concentrations (hyperglycaemia), elevated conversion of glucose into fat, and deposition of fat into central fat stores.

Insulin is the key regulating hormone that controls glucose uptake into the brain via its regulation of glutamine synthetase. As we have seen, insulin resistance is the major mechanism in modern humans that inhibits glucose transfer into the brain by its negative influence on glutamine synthetase. If oxytocin improves working memory, might this action result from positive oxytocin influence on insulin? It has indeed been shown that oxytocin positively affects several aspects of glucose regulation, including improved insulin sensitivity. A 2017 study in the journal *Diabetes* demonstrated that oxytocin acutely improved beta-cell responsiveness and glucose tolerance in healthy men.[60] So, oxytocin increases insulin sensitivity.

A trial published in the journal *Molecular Autism* in 2020 indicated that oxytocin's possible use in autism was indeed promising.[61] The authors concluded that oxytocin offered long-term beneficial effects for repetitive behaviours and feelings of avoidance.

## Vasopressin, oxytocin and the glutamatergic pathway

Bio-scientists often refer to glutamine synthetase and its regulation of glutamate and glutamine functions as the 'glutamatergic pathway'.

As we have seen, vasopressin and oxytocin modulate two of the most important homeostatic survival pathways in humans – hydration and energy. Late-modern refined-sugar-consuming humans are chronically energy and water stressed. Both vasopressin and oxytocin have been shown positively to influence cognition. We know that the glutamatergic pathway in the brain is central to cognitive facilitation and therefore also to impairment, so it is not surprising to discover that both hormones are involved in influencing this pathway.

A study, published in 2007 in the *Journal of Neurochemistry* by a team at the Department of Biomedical Sciences, Iowa State University, USA, showed that vasopressin positively influenced the glutamatergic pathway via increased glutamate release in the cerebral cortex.[62] Another study in the same year, published in the *Journal of Neuroscience* by a team from the Colleges of Medicine and Pharmacy at the University of Florida, USA, found that oxytocin receptors were expressed in glutamatergic prefrontal cortical neurones that modulate social recognition.[63]

# Raised blood glucose and the risk of metabolic disease

Before detailed consideration of each of the individual sugar sickness syndromes I would like to return to evidence that raised blood glucose, for whatever reason, is linked to metabolic disease. This link is confirmed when we look at whether the risk of developing obesity, type 2 diabetes, Alzheimer's disease and autism spectrum disorders is increased when hyperglycaemia is *not* the result of overconsumption of refined carbohydrates and sugars. Two such causes are viral hyperglycaemia (COVID-19 is an example) and insulin resistance due to urban air pollution.

These two environmental influences provide us with perfect control conditions to compare with the post-1970s increased consumption of refined carbohydrates and sugars. In each case it seems that blood glucose concentrations rise significantly, on the one hand driven by environmental influences such as pollution, and on the other by increased sugar consumption. If the sugar sickness syndromes are increased by each of these events, we can identify excess circulating glucose as a major, or *the* major, influence on the catastrophic decline in human health and cognition that is advancing around the world.

### Urban air pollution and the sugar sickness syndromes

Air pollution is known to be causing enormous health damage to humans around the world, including respiratory diseases, cancers, allergies, heart damage, irritation and deterioration of the eyes, nose and throat, reproductive harm, ailments in organs such as the gut, liver, spleen and blood, and extensive nervous system injuries. However, it is not normally considered in relation to the dysregulated energy and metabolic diseases that currently plague our species. These sugar sickness syndromes are usually associated with poor lifestyle and diet, and less so with other environmental influences. Nevertheless, there is evidence to suggest that air pollution can make us fat by negatively influencing energy-regulating systems in the human body.

In any organ or tissue supplied from the circulation, cell membranes are the protective layer that allows vital nutrients and essential molecules such as oxygen and energy to enter the cell, and waste products to exit. Cell membranes are highly complex and have multiple channels and pumping mechanisms that enable cells to carry out their main activities, and to maintain their housekeeping functions. Air-borne particulates interfere with these functions, damaging the cell and its mechanisms.

*Air pollution can cause obesity by negatively influencing our energy-regulation systems – particulates cause insulin resistance and inflammation leading to suppression of glutamine synthetase.*

When glucose is absorbed into the bloodstream from the gut, it requires insulin released from the pancreas to access the various tissues and the organs that it fuels. Studies have shown that exposure to particulate matter may induce increased blood glucose levels via several mechanisms, including insulin resistance, inflammation and vascular dysfunction. Increased blood glucose concentration will suppress glutamine synthetase and thereby inhibit glucose entry to the brain, leading to increased appetite and hunger, a scenario that would lead over time to obesity. If the initiating mechanism and sequence of events began with high levels of circulating glucose that is driven not by diet, but rather by air pollution, and this was followed by conversion of glucose to fats in an attempt to maintain stable blood glucose, we would have a mechanism that confirms that obesity is a glucose-driven condition, a sugar sickness syndrome.

To look at this from the opposite perspective, have each of the sugar sickness syndromes been shown to be associated with urban air pollution? There is evidence that this is indeed the case with obesity,[64] type 2 diabetes,[65] Alzheimer's disease[66] and autism spectrum disorders.[67]

## Viral hyperglycaemia and the sugar sickness syndromes

Viruses are sub-microscopic infectious agents. They replicate only inside living cells and infect all life forms in animal and plant organisms. They are 'clever' and commandeer the host cell machinery to replicate copies of themselves. They regularly mutate, a strategy to avoid the host immune system. Their viral 'intelligence' is such that they have no need to source their own energy supply and simply steal it from their hosts. In humans, they cause increased blood glucose concentration, often to dangerous levels. I have named this condition 'viral diabetes', a condition that has emerged as a major influence in Covid-19, and as a serious neurodegenerative manifestation in long-Covid.

*Viral infection causes hyperglycaemia that results in turn in inflammation and neurodegeneration.*

Viruses rarely cross the blood-brain barrier; the tightly controlled protective system prevents them from doing so. It may therefore be asked, if viruses do not enter the brain, how is it that they may initiate major neurodegenerative influences?

The answer is 'As a result of hyperglycaemia'. As is referenced throughout this book, hyperglycaemia oxidatively degrades the enzyme glutamine synthetase, the upstream mechanism that causes inflammation in microglia plus increased glutamate excitotoxicity, each of which contributes to neurone cytotoxicity and death. These downstream influences are driving forces in the four sugar sickness syndromes that I will now discuss in individual chapters, beginning with obesity.

## In summary...

The vital enzyme glutamine synthetase is suppressed by oxidation arising from high levels of insulin and sugar in the bloodstream.

This suppression is associated with the brain being starved of energy, oxygen and water. Our metabolic feedback systems tell us to consume more of these but they fail to reach our starving brains and the vicious cycle continues. This systemic problem is upstream of obesity, type 2 diabetes, Alzheimer's disease and autism spectrum disorders.

# Chapter 5

# Sugar sickness syndrome #1: Obesity

Fat is good. Humans love fat. Indeed, humans are fat, naturally fat, and naturally, healthily fat.

A healthy human adult stores between 20 and 40 per cent fat, depending on age and sex. Women are composed of higher levels of fat compared with men of similar age. This may be consistent with the energy demands of pregnancy and childbirth. A new child is born with a large package of body fat, a protective measure against potential maternal malnutrition.

Every cell in the body is surrounded by membranes that are composed of lipids (fats) that protect the cell and manage transmission of oxygen, energy, nutrients and other vital elements into it and waste out. Inside each cell is all the machinery required for life: DNA for replication and repair, proteins for growth and a host of organelles that do all the housekeeping and work of each cell, depending on which tissue or organ it is part of. Muscle cells 'contract', retinal cells 'see', olfactory cells 'smell', oral cells 'taste' and neurones 'think' or transmit electrical signals that we describe as thinking. Cell membranes are highly complex structures, consisting of a double phospholipid layer and containing multiple protein receptors that respond to a variety of information inputs, energy, nutrients, hormones and other factors, and to two-way signalling systems that maintain their health and function. Fats are an essential ingredient of cell membranes (they provide the 'lipids' in phospholipids) and therefore essential to life. And not only to life, but to cognition.

## Fats in human history

Our brains are composed of around 60% fat (lipids), and human brain cell membranes are composed of phospholipids that contain two vital fats, known as docosahexaenoic acid (DHA – an omega-3 fatty acid) and arachidonic acid (AA – an omega-6 fatty acid), without which cognition would not be possible. Our ancestors obtained these essential fats from meat and fish. Plant sources could not have supplied sufficient amounts of these fats for the development of our large brains and for the cognitive, communicative and linguistic advances that characterise our species.

One school of thought (known as the aquatic ape theory) suggests that our ancestors accessed marine, river and lake environments to obtain the necessary fats required to increase brain size and that we started out as a marine species.

We also know that without our ability as a species to efficiently utilise body fat storage capacity, we might not have survived the many periods of famine and starvation in our evolutionary history. We have the ability to run on short supply during periods of fasting and famine, we can break down body fat into small fat molecules, known as ketones, that the brain may use as a survival strategy. Our ability to fuel our bodies and brains with either glucose or fats contributes to our success in adapting to a huge range of environments. (Interestingly, cancer cells can be fuelled only by glucose, not ketones, but that is another story.)

Fats also made their contribution to the development of our advanced cognition, as a species. Humans have developed highly sophisticated sensory systems that enable them to recognise and access foods that are energy dense and nutritionally beneficial, and this contributed to the growth of a large, energy-expensive and cognitively advanced brain.

## Fats in the human brain

Around 60% of the brain is composed of fat with the remainder being made of a combination of water, protein, carbohydrates and salts. It also contains about 20% of the body's much-maligned cholesterol.

Omega-3 and omega-6 polyunsaturated fatty acids (PUFAs) are essential constituents of all cell membranes, allowing them to function as a selective barrier/gatekeeper for what goes in and out of cells. The omega-3s exhibit anti-inflammatory and neuroprotective properties and are thought to represent a potential treatment for a variety of neurodegenerative and neurological disorders. There are three involved in brain function: eicosapentaenoic acid (EPA), docosahexaenoic acid (DHA) and, more recently recognised, docosapentaenoic acid (DPA), each of which has unique effects. DHA in particular has a unique and indispensable role in neuronal membranes.

In addition, the axons of nerve cells rely for their lightning-speed transmission of electric signals on a fatty myelin sheath. Myelin contains high levels of saturated very-long-chain fatty acids derived from cholesterol and manufactured de novo (from scratch) in the brain by glia (astrocytes) and oligodendrocytes because cholesterol molecules are too large to cross the blood-brain barrier.

Without these two very different types of fat, the brain could not function.

## *Life without carbohydrates and sugars*

It is worth noting that, of the three macro-foods that humans consume, proteins and fats are essential to life and carbohydrates are not, and if the dietary sources available to humans consist only of these two foods, we can survive. We can run the brain on ketones if we have sufficient fat stores and we can manufacture glucose from proteins (a process known as gluconeogenesis that occurs in the liver).

It has indeed been proved that humans can survive without consuming carbohydrate foods. Vilhjalmur Stefansson was a famous Icelandic explorer, born in Canada of Icelandic extraction but who later became an American citizen. He had travelled extensively in the Arctic and had observed that the Inuit diet consisted almost exclusively of meat and fish for nine months of the year.

During a four-year expedition to the Canadian Arctic, Stefansson, along with a companion explorer, Dr Karsten Anderson, conducted research for the American Museum of Natural History, during which they lived off the land, eating only animal meat from kills and fish that they caught. Although they had taken so-called 'civilised' foods with them, they declined to eat these, and survived perfectly well on the food that was freely available from the local habitat. They returned to the metropolis in excellent health. Their dietary claims were met with much scepticism so they agreed to take part in a controlled study to prove what they had experienced in the Arctic. This study, over a year, became one of the most rigorous and famous dietary research projects in the history of nutritional science.[1] The authors were Walter S McClellan and Eugene F Du Bois. The investigation was monitored by an advisory group of scientists, of which the chairman was Dr Raymond Pearl of Johns Hopkins University, Baltimore. The work was conducted from the Russell Sage Institute of Pathology in Bellevue Hospital New York. The food was measured to the gram, so that there was no question of any dietary manipulation.

The key findings were:

- The two men lived on an exclusive meat diet with fat for one year.
- At the end of the year, they were both mentally alert, physically active and showed no specific physical changes in any system of the body.

It must be noted that the authors acknowledged that there was carbohydrate in the meat in the form of glycogen (glucose) stored in muscle to the extent of 7-12 grams per day. However, this could not have constituted a quantity of carbohydrate (as sugars) sufficient to negate the nature of the diet, and the explorers were vindicated in their claims.

## Hibernation and migration

Humans are not the only species to express sophisticated fat storage capacity. Many bird and animal species also do so, but in their case the fats play a particularly highly specialised role of providing the energy to fuel major life events, such as migration and hibernation.

**Migration**: Migrating birds for instance double their weight in two weeks, and fat is the added energy chosen for storage, before taking off on migratory flights over thousands of miles. Many researchers have debated why birds and animals (including marine species) migrate, but the simplest explanation makes most sense – animals migrate as a survival strategy. They leave one area where energy resources may be limited, in keeping with the energy required for growth and reproduction, and if the cost of migration is less than the energy gain in a new environment, migration is beneficial.

**Hibernation** is a strategy of dormancy and reduced metabolic rate during periods when food/energy resources are low, such as during the winter. Although this approach seems to be less energy dependent compared to the high cost of migration, in so far as less energy is being expended, the time may be extended over several months, and therefore the total energy stored and required for that period may be significantly greater than for migration. Female polar bears give birth during hibernation, and this represents a colossal extra energy burden. Cubs must be fed via lactation. The mothers lose lean tissue; brown bears may lose up to 70% of their lean tissues in the winter months.

## Widespread obesity is a new condition

For most of the history and prehistory of humans, the acquisition and consumption of the necessary energy resources to maintain all the functions of life, including reproduction of new generations, has been the major goal and influence on behaviour. Prior to the domestication of plants and animals when the human population was much smaller, our hunter-gatherer ancestors appear usually to have been well provisioned (see page 14), except in the more weather-extreme regions of the world.

After the introduction of farming, food production rapidly increased, along with the population, but that dividend was subject to weather and pestilence, and was always vulnerable. Famines were a regular hazard. As civilisation developed, adequate food resources became more associated with the ruling strata in society, and classes evolved that could expropriate these at the expense of others.

Obesity, a condition of energy accumulation, is not new, but until the 20th century was associated almost exclusively with power and prosperity. Malnutrition was universal around the world, and hunger was still a major health concern in the USA as late as the 1960s.

## Fats good: Obesity bad

If fats are so essential to life, why is having too much stored fat so bad? These are the official risks and outcomes of obesity sourced from the UK's NHS and the USA Department of Health and Human Services:

- type 2 diabetes
- heart disease
- stroke
- high blood pressure
- elevated cholesterol
- sleep apnoea
- arthritis
- some cancers
- infertility.

Do note that the brain and neurodegeneration are not directly referenced as in any way connected with obesity initiation or progression in this official list. The notion of neurodegenerative damage and shrinkage of the brain is absent, but the aim of this book is to show that these are the most important consequences and that we can still do something about this. As I have shown, the upstream cause of obesity is in the brain, and is driven by chronic brain-energy depletion, making obesity a neurological disease. All the other effects specified in the list are downstream from that single event – oxidative suppression of the enzyme glutamine synthetase, the human brain's fuel pump, by excess sugar consumption.

### The official causes of obesity

With glutamine synthetase suppression not in the picture, what then are the official reasons given for the rise in obesity? The following have been taken from the UK's NHS and the USA National Institutes of Health sources. (The US Centers for Disease Control and Prevention (CDC) did suggest avoiding food and beverages high in sugar.)

- Eating a poor diet of foods high in fats and calories.

- Having a sedentary (inactive) lifestyle.
- Not sleeping enough, which can lead to hormonal changes that make you feel hungrier and crave certain high-calorie foods.
- Genetics, which can affect how your body processes food into energy and how fat is stored.
- The 'ageing population'/growing older, which can lead to less muscle mass and a slower metabolic rate, making it easier to gain weight.
- Pregnancy (weight gained during pregnancy can be difficult to lose and may eventually lead to obesity).

Do note that sugars are not referenced in any of these 'causes'. I could not find them listed on any of the websites except that recommendation by CDC to avoid high sugars.

## Obesity: The true cause

We know what causes obesity – excess consumption of refined carbohydrates and sugars. We know because obesity has exploded globally in a few decades consistent with the increased consumption of sugars from the 1970s on. The ground-breaking paper by Grasgruber and colleagues (2018) cites 'Muslim countries which simultaneously consume the highest amount of cereals and wheat in the world and suffer from very high obesity rates'.[2]

Fat consumption in that period has not significantly increased as we saw in Chapter 1 and this is largely because fats have been removed from processed foods and sugars added. According to Robert Lustig, a leading anti-refined sugar academic, processed foods now constitute up to 80% of the US diet, and the UK is not far behind. Yes, we may eat excess calories over those we spend, but these calories consist mostly of refined carbohydrates and sugars that rapidly release excess glucose into the circulation and suppress the brain's energy pump.

*Figure 3: Trends in sugar consumption and obesity from 1960 to now*

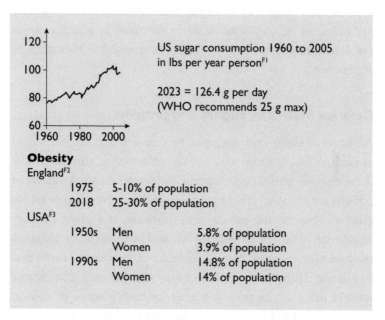

120
100
80
60
1960 1980 2000

US sugar consumption 1960 to 2005 in lbs per year person[F1]

2023 = 126.4 g per day (WHO recommends 25 g max)

**Obesity**
England[F2]

| | | |
|---|---|---|
| | 1975 | 5-10% of population |
| | 2018 | 25-30% of population |
| USA[F3] | | |
| | 1950s | Men | 5.8% of population |
| | | Women | 3.9% of population |
| | 1990s | Men | 14.8% of population |
| | | Women | 14% of population |

## Is a calorie simply a calorie?

One of the paradoxes of obesity is that people with large fat stores feel permanently hungry. All sorts of theories around hormones have been proposed. One of the most ludicrous reasons given for obesity is that it is simply a case of eating or consuming more calories than we spend. According to this theory all calories are the same, and therefore reducing them to food type is foolish. Really?

Bombs consist of mega quantities of explosive fuel calories, which are released in one colossal metabolic event. If a large bomb was in the form of a giant chocolate cake, consisting of the same number of calories as a smaller and real bomb, such as a hand grenade, and was dropped onto the ground from a great height, would the result be the same? Unlikely; the chocolate calories would have been provided in a form that was not inherently explosive, no matter how efficient the charge, and if people were around, they might be splurged with chocolate, but probably not killed by an explosion. Clearly the form in which calories are delivered in any energy system, mechanical or biological, is significant.

### Calories from fats, sugars and proteins

A calorie of sugar (glucose) may be converted to fat and stored as such. A calorie of fat may not be converted to glucose – there is no enzyme pathway in human biology to do so. A calorie of protein may be converted to glucose and therefore also to fat via glucose. Assume the human diet consisted of a given number of calories of fat (F), of glucose (G) and of protein (P). Humans may survive on an FP diet – a protein portion may be converted to glucose. Humans theoretically may survive on a glucose and protein diet (GP) because a portion of both glucose or protein may be converted to fat. However, no survival is possible on a glucose and fat diet (FG) because neither glucose nor fat may be converted to protein (neither fats nor glucose contain nitrogen, the essential element of amino acids). The notion that a calorie is a calorie independent of food type is therefore nonsense.

Furthermore, the three macro-nutrients have very different 'thermic effects' – the amount of energy needed for your body to digest, absorb and metabolise a food. If you consume 100 fat calories, only 3 calories are spent digesting the fat so you get 97 per cent of the energy. Carbohydrates have a thermic effect of 5-10 per cent and proteins, a thermic effect of 30 per cent.

## Is obesity a condition of calorie imbalance or calorie 'partition'?

To understand why excess sugars lead to increased fat stores but continuing hunger, consider this scenario:

## Chapter 5

If we take two healthy subjects, one consuming total energy intake as refined sugar and the other the same total energy intake in the form of honey.

Assume that the human body consists of just two separate chambers (body and brain), with a given total energy input of, say, 2500 calories in 24 hours.

We know the brain burns around 150 grams of glucose in 24 hours – that is, 600 calories. Therefore, the other 1900 calories will be provided ('partitioned') to the body to be used for metabolism, locomotion etc; excess will be stored in the liver and muscles as glycogen for easy access and any excess beyond that will be stored as fat.

If the theory 'calories in/out' is correct, the proportion partitioned to the body would be the same in both individuals, and the quantity retained as body fat should also be the same.

However, if the glucose calories are derived from refined sugars and blood glucose concentration rises, the excess will be oxidised and suppress the enzyme glutamine synthetase; glucose will consequently not be pumped across the blood-brain barrier, and this will deprive the brain of energy. In these circumstances, where will the surplus glucose calories that are not entering the hungry brain now go? They will be converted to fat under the influence of insulin and stored in the body's fat (adipose) tissue.

If the total sugar calories are supplied as honey, something different occurs. The battery of antioxidant bioflavonoids in the honey will protect the enzyme glutamine synthetase from oxidation, its role as the brain's fuel pump will be facilitated and the glucose required by the brain will be efficiently transferred (pumped) into the brain by that enzyme. Less will be partitioned to the body and stored as fat.

As these alternatives demonstrate, the 'partition' of calories (the basis on which they are divided between body and brain) with the two types of sugar is different. In the case of refined sugars, the brain is deprived of energy, and more energy is stored in the body in the form of fat calories – the body grows at the expense of the brain. In the case of the honey eaters, the bioflavonoids will prevent oxidation of glutamine synthetase, allowing the enzyme to pump the calories required to maintain brain function, based exclusively on its fuel demand.

*Too much sugar suppresses the brain's energy pump so the brain fails to get the energy it craves, increasing hunger.*

Fewer calories will be available to the body, and less fat will be deposited. In each case, the partition of the energy is different, and the outcomes are different. Therefore, the notion that obesity is simply a result of calorie imbalance is incorrect. (NB The same would occur if the calories were supplied as fat: glutamine synthetase would not be suppressed so the brain would get the energy it needed.)

Think of it this way. A physician believes the calories in/out perspective. A patient is diagnosed with obesity and type 2 diabetes. The physician explains to the patient that they must exercise and eat fewer calories. However, the same physician also prescribes metformin to combat the type 2 diabetes. Why? If the calories in/out hypothesis were correct, this physician would be acting counter to their philosophy. Reduction of calories intake alone would solve the problem.

As it happens, the antidiabetic medication metformin, now being recommended in obesity, partitions glucose to the brain by upgrading the enzyme glutamine synthetase, thereby reducing blood glucose concentration and the conversion of circulating glucose calories to fat.[3] In other words, a proportion of the incoming calories has been diverted to the brain and not converted to fat. This confused physician believes in the calories in/out perspective but behaves as a metabolic philosopher of partition and offers a drug that diverts blood glucose into the brain, thereby preventing its conversion to fat in the body. As you can see, metformin acts in the same fashion as does honey, via the honey bioflavonoids – in the brain.

## The neurology of weight gain

Obesity is a disease of high energy consumption in the form of sugars and refined carbohydrates that deliver excess glucose into the circulation. Excess circulating glucose impairs the functioning of the human brain's fuel pump, causing brain energy deprivation and increased brain hunger. Appetite hormones are released. The cycle repeats. The excess energy is converted to fats and stored under the influence of insulin, the sugar-regulating hormone. Every other negative effect associated with obesity follows downstream from that mechanism – the body grows fatter at the expense of the brain.

Although obesity was well researched in the latter part of the 20th century, little sense of its origins in, and damage inflicted on, the brain emerged until the early 21st century. For this change, we must thank Antonio Convit MD, at the Department of Psychiatry, New York University, USA, who, as a Professor of Psychiatry, Medicine and Radiology, has focused on the impact of obesity and obesity-associated metabolic dysregulation, including type 2 diabetes, on cognitive functions and brain structural integrity.

In November 2010, Antonio Convit and colleagues published a study in the journal *Diabetologia* that first raised the alarm that obesity might have significant damaging effects on the human brain.[4] Earlier studies had implicated type 2 diabetes in brain damage, but this was the first to implicate obesity. Perhaps even more alarming was the news that the study was conducted in adolescents; they were obese and had type 2 diabetes.

What of obese adolescents who did not have type 2 diabetes? In 2011, Professor Convit and colleagues published a study in the journal *Obesity* that addressed that question.[5] The authors examined obese adolescents whose eating was uncontrolled ('disinhibited') and the conclusions were alarming: they found 'that relative to lean adolescents, obese participants had lower performance on cognitive tests, and lower orbitofrontal cortex volume'.

*Obesity has been shown to be associated with brain shrinkage in areas associated with cognition and decision making.*

This was a devastating conclusion. The orbitofrontal cortex is an area involved in cognition and decision making. Here was the first indication that obesity is a condition that may involve shrinkage of the human brain in adolescents. Why were the alarm bells not rung everywhere childhood obesity was already a recognised and growing problem?

## The shrinking brain

Why, if the condition of brain reduction had already been recognised in obese type 2 diabetics, were sugars not recognised as the most likely perpetrator? If parents had been alerted that excess consumption of sugars, in beverages, foods and snacks, might/could/would shrink the brains of their children, would their views about food consumption not have changed? It is not possible to know the answer because the alarm bells were never rung.

Have you, the reader, ever encountered an overweight or obese individual who was conscious of the neurodegenerative effects of overweight or obesity, or that these conditions might shrink the human brain? Have you ever encountered an overweight or obese individual who was conscious that every gram of overweight accumulation constituted a symptom of potential brain energy that had been diverted and stored in the body? Have you ever encountered a physician or other health professional who articulated just this as a scientific hypothesis, or as a potential scientific conclusion?

Have the National Institutes of Health in the US, or one of the equivalents around the world, ever issued a statement to the effect that overweight and obesity are conditions of reduced brain energy provision, and therefore a mechanism for reduced brain volume? I suspect your answer will be 'No' on each and every count.

## What bariatric surgery tells us about blood glucose, weight loss and cognition

Bariatric (weight loss) surgery includes a variety of gastric bypass interventions that modulate the gut so that the intake of food and calories is reduced. Bariatric procedures have proved to be highly effective in reducing weight and improving health outcomes, such as cardiovascular risks. The American National Institutes of Health reported in 2013 that there was a 29% reduction in mortality for those who undertook the procedure.[6] However, back in 1995 a team from the School of Medicine and Human Performance Laboratory at East Carolina University, USA,[7] had described bariatric surgery not simply as effective in treating type 2 diabetes, but as the *most effective* treatment. It seems an outrageous conclusion – how can it be possible to operate on a condition of high circulating blood glucose levels? It certainly is not possible to surgically enter the blood vessels and extract the excess glucose.

Of Americans who are diabetic, 90% have type 2 diabetes. The various therapies used to treat the condition, including insulin, oral antidiabetic drugs, diet and exercise, are not usually successful in totally controlling blood glucose levels. The incidence of complications such as stroke, heart disease, kidney failure, blindness, gangrene and cognitive decline continue to pose major health challenges.

The authors were able to report that their surgical interventions in obese diabetic patients with poorly controlled blood glucose levels, restored and maintained normal levels of glucose and insulin, for up to 14 years, a much higher degree of diabetic control than any other medical strategy. However, the most significant finding was that blood glucose concentrations were reduced within days of the procedure, *long before weight loss kicked in*. The weight loss was a downstream event, secondary to the lowered blood glucose concentration. This has significant implications for our understanding of the relationship between obesity and type 2 diabetes.

### Obesity: Disguised diabetes?

We usually consider that weight gain and obesity precede the development of type 2 diabetes, and that is the trajectory for most people; indeed, physicians invariably warn their obese patients of their high risk of developing type 2 diabetes. If we travel upstream and include the brain, a different perspective emerges. Excess circulating glucose suppresses the brain's fuel pump, depriving the brain of energy and the hungry brain activates the appetite hormones stimulating the consumption of more sugar; the cycle repeats. The glucose that cannot be pumped across the blood-brain barrier is retained in the bloodstream, and if superfluous to requirements, is converted to fat and stored under the influence of insulin. As described above, the accumulated fat is therefore potential brain energy that has been stolen by the body. The body gains energy at the expense of the brain.

In this perspective, weight gain is a form of early diabetes –

but *disguised* because the excess circulating glucose is converted to fat – it is taken out of the bloodstream so blood sugar levels remain 'normal'. Of course, a portion of the weight gain will also consist of dietary fat, which has been stored, but that mechanism is driven by insulin and insulin is primarily a sugar regulatory hormone. As I have said before, dietary fat consumption has not significantly increased over the last half century; that particularly toxic dietary prize has been well and truly won by refined carbohydrates and sugars.

## Bariatric surgery, blood sugar control and cognition

If the generating influence in weight gain begins with impaired glucose uptake by the brain and consequent neurodegenerative damage, we should look to see whether bariatric surgery exerts a potential positive influence on cognition.

In 2016 a combined team from the Universities of Wales and Swansea, UK, examined the effect of weight loss resulting from bariatric surgery on cognitive function.[8] They reviewed data from 18 earlier publications, and their conclusions were striking. They: 'noted significant and rapid weight loss resulting from bariatric surgery is associated with prompt and sustained improvements in cognitive function including memory, executive function, and cognitive control.'

In other words, bariatric surgery links together three sugar sickness syndromes: obesity, type 2 diabetes and Alzheimer's disease.

## Rapamycin and the mTOR pathway

Easter Island is an Oceanic Island, famous for its ancient *moai* statues. It may seem unlikely that we would connect Easter Island, an island with important historical information on environmental damage inflicted by human habitation, with modern environmental influences on human energy dynamics.

There is a link, however, and a significant one. Humans are notorious for their neglect of basic environmental hygiene with respect to Mother Earth. Easter Island has also proved to be important in improving our understanding of energy hygiene and of the potential damage to our own organism, in addition to that of the Earth.

In 1975 a new antifungal medication was discovered in the soil of Easter Island and named rapamycin after the native name *Rapa Nui*. Later work showed that this compound had significant anticancer potential and immunosuppressive properties and was developed into a successful medication to reduce organ rejection during transplant operations.

Gradually, and over many years, the complex actions of this interesting molecule were unravelled, and it emerged that rapamycin inhibited high-energy pathways in the human body. The major such pathway is known as the 'mammalian target of rapamycin' (mTOR) pathway, but in this book, we can use the term the 'sugar/insulin pathway', or perhaps better still, the 'ice/cream pathway', because this pathway regulates sugars and fats via insulin signalling and thereby:

- increases conversion of sugars to fats
- increases storage of these fats
- increases storage of dietary fats
- prevents stored fat from being released and burned
- drives the development of obesity, and obesity in turn activates this pathway
- also drives type 2 diabetes, Alzheimer's disease and autism.

Of particular interest is the understanding that the primary influence on the mTOR pathway may be in the brain.

In March 2013, Michael Wong of the Department of Neurology, Washington University, USA, published a study in the *Biomedical Journal* that opened a valuable window onto the action of this molecule in the brain and how it may improve neuropathological conditions.[9] Modern humans overconsume refined carbohy-drates and sugars and live in a state of chronic over-activation of this pathway. They therefore suffer the consequences in conditions such as obesity, type 2 diabetes, Alzheimer's disease and autism. Rapamycin opposes these actions and, by doing so, shows us the driving mechanisms underpinning each of the sugar sickness syndromes. Medications based on rapamycin are now being investigated as potential anti-obesity solutions.[10]

## The fat/thin/'fat' paradox of obesity and cognition

Obesity is a significant recognised risk factor for Alzheimer's disease. Combined with type 2 diabetes it is a higher risk factor still. This is not surprising because, as we have seen, high levels of circulating glucose suppress the enzyme glutamine synthetase, deprive the brain of energy and increase levels of toxic glutamate in the brain, which damages neurones. This simple description further suggests that these conditions share a common underlying pathway and cause.

Most of us will know of Alzheimer's patients who are not obese and may never have been. Indeed, Alzheimer's disease and other later life dementias are often associated with weight loss. Also, a higher late-life body mass index (BMI) indicating weight gain has been associated with some degree of protection against dementia, and Alzheimer's disease specifically. How can these seemingly contradictory findings be reconciled?

In 2014 a team from the Department of Neurobiology at the Karolinska Institute, in Stockholm, Sweden, reviewed this question in a study published by the *European Journal of Clinical Nutrition*.[11] and found that overweight and obesity were indeed linked to increased future dementia risk in old age. However, when examined in old age, a higher BMI was associated with better cognition and decreased mortality.

Although this finding may seem counterintuitive, there is actually a very simple explanation. Obesity at any age impairs cognition. That is now well established and no longer controversial though not widely talked about. The fundamental and upstream mechanism for this effect is that obesity via excess circulating glucose and oxidative degradation of glutamine synthetase results in loss of energy supply to the brain. In other words, when the body is over-supplied with energy the brain is under-supplied, so excess body fat is an index of potential dementia.

This paradoxical condition mimics the state of energy deficiency in famine and starvation. The brain reacts as it would in such an emergency – it degrades body tissues to create new glucose. The tissues selected are proteins, mainly from muscle. These are taken to the liver and converted to glucose, and released into the circulation, adding to the initial problem. Weight is being lost, but this weight is not fat. It is muscle.

Muscle tissue is expensive to maintain in terms of energy, and it uses up glucose, consequently that protection is also lost. Here we have an explanation of how dementia and Alzheimer's disease specifically, may be associated with weight loss in later life, a well-known phenomenon.

*Not all weight loss is positive – if it arises from muscle loss this is a risk factor for hyperglycaemia as the storage capacity for excess sugar is reduced.*

Body mass index (BMI) is a not a measure of the relative ratios of fat and lean tissue. In old age, a higher BMI which includes retained muscle tissue would offer some level of protection by reducing circulating glucose and freeing up the brain's fuel pump – the enzyme glutamine synthetase. In the fat/thin/fat narrative, the last and so-called protective contribution to body weight may actually consist of lean tissue, hidden within the BMI

measure, that offers some protection against neurodegeneration.
So with regard to weight regulation we know these facts about
the sugar sickness syndromes:

- Alzheimer's disease and weight regulation are intimately
  interconnected.
- Alzheimer's disease is a condition of impaired cognition,
  communication and language in later life.
- Autism is a condition of impaired cognition,
  communication and language starting in early life.

This raises questions about how obesity may also be interconnected with autism spectrum disorders.

### Obesity and autism: Is there a link?

Obesity is an energy dysregulated condition that is associated
with, and driven by, excess glucose in the human circulation, as
we have seen. This perspective does not exclude the view that fats
also contribute to obesity – they do, but under the influence of
insulin, a hormone that is largely released in response to glucose
(sugar), and not significantly to fats. In babies, obesity is a post-
birth condition, and the term does not apply to energy regulation
or dysregulation in the foetus. However, if energy dysregulation
does occur in the foetus due to maternal over-nutrition, and later
in infants and children during post-birth growth, it is highly
likely that the pre- and post-birth conditions may share energy
pathways and mechanisms that provide important information
about both autism and obesity. Is the mTOR high-energy pathway active in the cognitive impairments associated with autism?

In 2021 a major international study by a team from Italy,
Cyprus, Spain, America and the UK answered this question
decisively, in the journal *Nature Communications*.[12] The authors
established a mechanistic link between mTOR-related synaptic
pathology and autism, finding that aberrations in synaptic

pruning (an essential step in neurodevelopment) might lead to behavioural disruptions via alterations in neural connectivity.

Autism spectrum disorders in children as a recognised risk factor for weight gain had already been established in 2019 in a study published in the journal *Pediatric Obesity Review*.[13] Those authors analysed data from 35 studies published between 1999 and 2014 which examined increased weight or obesity in children diagnosed with autism spectrum disorders. Their conclusions were astonishing – they found that children with this diagnosis had a 41% increased risk of obesity compared with neurotypical children, and that obesity developed as early as 2 to 5 years of age. If glutamine synthetase is impaired during foetal development, the early developing brain is chronically deprived of energy and the appetite hormones are potentially over-activated, as is the case in adult-onset obesity.

If weight gain and obesity are directly related to autism spectrum disorders, a condition of impaired cognition, it may be expected that sugars would be that link, and that dysregulated insulin metabolism would be an influence.

### Insulin resistance, hyperinsulinaemia and brain energy in obesity

As you know, insulin is the hormone that promotes glucose transport into cells, thereby controlling blood glucose levels. Insulin resistance is a condition in which cells fail to respond to insulin, causing more and more insulin to be produced in an effort to stop blood glucose concentrations from rising. It is associated with excess consumption of refined carbohydrates and sugars. When cell membranes fail to efficiently transport glucose into the cells, the pancreas produces and releases more insulin to compensate for the resistance and the resulting hyperinsulinaemia is also unhealthy, increasing blood pressure and posing an additional risk of heart problems.

A 2000 study in the *Journal of Clinical Investigation*,[14] by researchers at Harvard Medical School, USA, looked into the relationship between obesity, insulin resistance and hyper-insulinaemia. The authors discovered that insulin resistance and hyperinsulinaemia, in addition to being caused by obesity, might contribute to its development – another vicious cycle driven by high levels of circulating glucose.

# Chapter 6

# Sugar sickness syndrome #2: Type 2 diabetes

Diabetes has been recognised since ancient times: it was described in an Egyptian document in 1500 BCE as a 'too great emptying of the urine'. The sweet urine associated with diabetes was known to the ancient Chinese, Indians, Greeks, Romans and Persians. It is a condition where blood sugar levels rise too high and the body attempts to flush this excess sugar out, resulting in extreme thirst and the constant need to urinate (polyuria), with the urine full of sugar. Until very recently it was endemic, at a relatively low level, but there has been an unprecedented rise in cases of type 2 diabetes since the 1970s, coinciding with the change to 'low-fat/high-carb' dietary guidelines. The World Health Organization (WHO) reported in 2016 that the increase in type 2 diabetes since 1980 had quadrupled and reached more than 400 million adults worldwide.[1]

Sarah Wild and colleagues, reporting in the journal *Diabetes Care* in May 2004 stated that worldwide the prevalence was 2.8% of the world's population in 2000 and would be 4.4% in 2030 – 171 million rising to 366 million at a very conservative estimate.[2]

In 2017, author Paul Zimmet described this as the 'diabesity epidemic' (obesity and type 2 diabetes), predicting it was likely to be the biggest epidemic in human history – with greater consequences than the Black Death in the 14th century and associated with epigenetic changes transmitted 'inter-generationally'.[3]

*Figure 4: Trends in sugar consumption and Type 2 diabetes from 1960 to now*

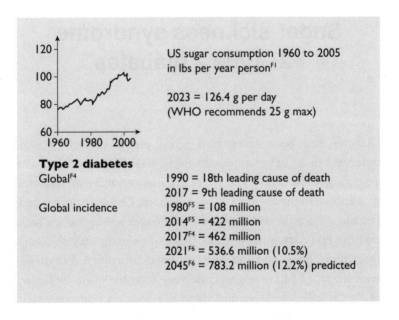

US sugar consumption 1960 to 2005 in lbs per year person[F1]

2023 = 126.4 g per day
(WHO recommends 25 g max)

**Type 2 diabetes**
Global[F4]

1990 = 18th leading cause of death
2017 = 9th leading cause of death

Global incidence

1980[F5] = 108 million
2014[F5] = 422 million
2017[F4] = 462 million
2021[F6] = 536.6 million (10.5%)
2045[F6] = 783.2 million (12.2%) predicted

## Type 1 and type 2 diabetes: What is the difference?

In the early years of the 20th century, two intrepid young researchers, John Rennie and Thomas Fraser at Aberdeen University, were to be viewed every morning in the cold winter months at Aberdeen Harbour on Scotland's north-east coast, where they were seeking a particular species of fish, *Lophius piscatorius* (popularly known as the monkfish), a fish that was distinguished by its unusually large and accessible pancreas, such that the pancreatic tissue could be easily removed.[4] The pancreas is the gland that produces and releases several important energy- and glucose-regulating hormones, including insulin. After a meal, insulin directs energy in the form of glucose into cells that require it to function. If insulin is absent or its function impaired, blood glucose concentration rises (hyperglycaemia) and the resulting condition is described as diabetes.

There are two major types of diabetes. Type 1 is a condition in which insulin is not produced by the pancreas and blood glucose rises to dangerous levels. This condition is thought to be largely autoimmune in origin, linked in some cases to infection and in others to food allergies/intolerances that lead to autoimmune destruction of the pancreas, but with a strong genetic component. Type 1 is also therefore referred to as 'insulin-dependent diabetes' and, before the introduction of insulin 100 years ago, most sufferers had a short life expectancy and died in ketoacidosis, though there were exceptions (see box).

---

### Treating type 1 diabetes with diet

JM and J Brostoff (both medical doctors) describe how their great/grandfather, who developed acute onset (type 1) diabetes in 1909, at the age of 29, 'survived by diet alone, aided by strength of will, for 14 years' until he could become one of the first patients in the UK to receive insulin, in August 1923. He had been given no more than four years to live. His strict diet was originally prescribed for him by the Kaiser's physician in Berlin and consisted of a dramatically reduced carbohydrate content but greatly increased fat. 'He was advised to eat fried bacon because it was high in fat.' This helped but his health slowly deteriorated so he tried something called the Allen diet that restricted calories to 1000 kcal per day; this kept him alive but barely able to function and he had to give up his work as a tailor. Then in 1916 he was given a new diet by Dr Otto Leyton that was 'absolutely sugar-free'. (Note that an Inuit 'ketogenic' diet includes 15% carbohydrates.) From 1918 onwards he

---

'maintained the low-energy diet... His weight fell from 82 to 64 kg as a result of the meagre diet but he managed to keep working'. He struggled on, including visiting the Bad Neuenahr spa, but was hardly more than skin and bones by the time insulin became available. Treatment with insulin at the London Hospital under the care of Otto Leyton completely turned things around and he lived healthily to the age of 88. His descendants say 'He was meticulous in the control of his blood sugar and gave himself more than 47,000 injections during his lifetime'.[5]

Type 2 diabetes does not cause, but rather results from, blood glucose levels being dangerously high, and is largely due to overconsumption of refined carbohydrates and sugars. In other words, type 1 *causes* high blood glucose levels; type 2 *is caused by* high blood glucose levels. These are two very different conditions, although superficially similar in terms of symptoms. Most of the world's diabetics have type 2, and it is this condition that has dramatically increased in numbers from the 1970s on.

## Establishing the role of insulin

Late in the 19th century, two German researchers, Oskar Minkowski and Josef von Mering, worked together at the University of Strasbourg on diabetes. They induced diabetes in dogs by removing the pancreas, thereby confirming the link between pancreatic function and blood glucose regulation and control. This critical finding was the catalyst for the work of the two intrepid young researchers, John Rennie and Thomas Fraser at Aberdeen University.

Rennie and Fraser were seeking to find and isolate a group of pancreatic cells known as the 'islets of Langerhans' which were believed to be the source of the substance that controlled blood glucose concentrations. They were successful in their efforts and supplied a raw or boiled extract to four diabetic patients, with some success in reducing blood glucose concentrations. However, due to supply problems and to the unpleasantness of the preparation, the patients died. Nevertheless, this was an historic and vital study and confirmed the role of the pancreas in blood glucose control. Their work influenced John James Rickard MacLeod, a Scottish biochemist from Aberdeen, who emigrated to America and later Canada, and eventually received the 1923 Nobel Prize for his work in discovering insulin, along with Frederik Banting, a Canadian researcher who worked in Macleod's laboratory at the University of Toronto.

As the work of these pioneering researchers showed, the pancreas is the gland that produces and releases several important energy- and glucose-regulating hormones, including insulin.

## Regulating our blood sugar levels

After a meal, when levels of glucose in blood plasma rise, insulin directs glucose into the organs and tissues that require it for use as energy. If there is more than immediately needed, insulin directs excess glucose into the two energy storage facilities, muscle and the liver, where it is stored as glycogen, a kind of concentrated human starch. Between meals and overnight the liver releases glucose into the bloodstream, essentially to supply the brain. The muscle store, although much larger than the liver, is reserved exclusively for movement and locomotion and is not available to the brain; muscle cells do not contain the special enzymes (glycogen phosphorylase and glycogen branching enzyme) that release glucose back into the circulation.

In our history as hunter gatherers, it was important to have glucose available for intense physical exercise, to hunt prey or escape from a predator. Muscles do use fats to fuel locomotion, but only at a low level of activity, such as walking or slow-paced running; during acute physical motion only glucose can rapidly fuel increases in power output, a vital survival system in dangerous situations. Reserving a readily available, and easily mobilised, energy store in muscle was a vital survival strategy. A modern athlete will use virtually no fats in a sprint.

If during a prolonged and intense physical event, such as a marathon, when muscle glucose stores become depleted, contracting muscles are obliged to extract glucose from the circulation; at this stage they are therefore using the brain's fuel reserve. In other words, the two tissues (brain and muscle) compete for fuel, and it is not surprising that many athletes collapse at this point. If the liver reserve is low, the brain simply aborts the enterprise, or if the athlete staggers on to the finish, he or she is often incoherent due to lack of brain energy supply.

### Glucose and the liver: Claude Bernard

Claude Bernard was a French physician and physiologist who lived from 1813 to 1878 and is rightly considered to be one of the greatest life-scientists of all time. In his laboratory in Paris, he contributed historic work on diabetes, and probably his most important contribution was that he established the major role played by the liver in the condition. In his early work he established that digestion of cane sugar and starch resulted in the release of absorbable glucose in the gut. Later he discovered glucose in the circulation, and that in all animal livers he examined there were significant quantities of glucose, a finding that was as unexpected as it was revelatory. He also observed that glucose appeared in the circulation in humans who had been fasting for several days, suggesting that the human body could synthesise it.

Bernard proved that the liver could store glucose, in a form which he described as glycogen, and that this was under the control of the brain via the nervous system. We now understand that the small liver glycogen store is the only reserve store of energy available to the brain between meals and during the overnight fast. In one famous experiment he took an animal liver that they had previously analysed for its glucose content, and that had been left overnight by an assistant. He found that there was more glucose in the liver than was the case on the previous day. This was a stunning finding and proved for the first time that the liver could manufacture glucose, as had been suggested in the earlier fasting experiment; it did not, however, indicate the source of the new glucose.[6]

We now know humans can break down protein to glucose through the process of gluconeogenesis.

## Regulating the fuel supply to our brain

By the beginning of the 20th century, researchers had developed a preliminary idea of how human energy intake, 'partition' (division between parts of the organism needing it) and regulation were organised. Bernard had shown that the liver stored and manufactured glucose. Importantly he had also shown that this was under the control of the brain via the nervous system. Oskar Minkowski had demonstrated that the pancreas was an important player in this process, and that absence of the gland resulted in increased blood glucose levels. Rennie and Fraser, had likewise demonstrated that some principle within the pancreas was able to exert control of glucose concentration in the bloodstream.

The next question puzzling researchers was how did the brain exert its control over the release of glucose from the liver. We know today that if blood glucose concentration falls, the brain is immediately at risk and organises the release of glucose from the liver, via the breakdown of glycogen. How does it do this?

## Adrenaline and the stress response

In 1903, at the Laboratory of the Royal College of Physicians in Edinburgh, Scotland, the question was brilliantly answered by D Noel Paton, a Scottish physician and academic, who was Regus Professor of Physiology at the University of Glasgow. Paton injected adrenaline into animals with and without pancreases and painted adrenaline onto the pancreases of live animals (through a complicated process) and found that blood glucose concentrations rose, and that glucose appeared in the urine, a classic description of diabetes.[7] He also noted that proteins were being degraded and that production of ammonia increased, both of which are characteristic of protein breakdown and the release of nitrogen.

From Bernard it was known that the liver could manufacture glucose and Paton's work pointed to proteins as the source of the new glucose, and that the hormone adrenaline was involved. Injecting or painting adrenaline mimicked the production of adrenaline during physical stress. However, *in this case the action was at rest*, and therefore mimicked sedentary stress, characteristic of modern sedentary humans. Paton's work should not be underestimated; he showed that if the brain was deprived of energy over time, it would degrade protein to make glucose in the liver. *In other words, the brain eats the body*.

We now understand that Paton was describing the stress response that always occurs when the brain is at risk of losing its fuel supply. Adrenaline releases glucose from the liver glycogen store and cortisol causes proteins to be degraded and transported to the liver to make new glucose, although at the time cortisol was not known. This response of the brain is popularly known as the fight-or-flight response, but this description is only partially correct.

Although the response to a threat leads to increased glucose in the bloodstream, its primary role is to protect the brain. Contracting muscles extract glucose from the circulation, deplete the liver and place the brain at risk of running out of fuel. The brain responds by releasing stores of glucose to ensure its continuing fuel supply and, if necessary, creating new glucose from degraded protein as back up. Modern athletes who fail to fuel correctly and over-train, chronically stimulate their adrenals and degrade their muscle protein, a major health hazard.

## The high blood glucose/hungry brain paradox

It may seem paradoxical that in the case of Paton's unfortunate animals, who were certainly sedentary, that the brain activated protein breakdown when the glucose supply was already high, as is the case in diabetes. Why was this? The answer is that the additional glucose in the circulation *prevented* glucose from gaining access to the brains of Paton's animals and the mechanism for this was the oxidation and degradation of the enzyme glutamine synthetase, as described in earlier chapters, driven by high levels of sugar in the blood.

Modern humans consume excess refined carbohydrates and sugars, a new event in our evolutionary history. This results first in chronically raised levels of insulin and, as the body's response to insulin fails, in chronically elevated blood glucose concentrations, in some cases associated with obesity and prediabetes/metabolic syndrome, and in others with type 2 diabetes. Excess circulating glucose suppresses the enzyme glutamine synthetase, directly and via excess insulin.

As described in Chapter 2, this essential enzyme acts as the brain's fuel pump as part of the glutamine/glutamate cycle (see page 36). The higher the glucose concentration, the more pronounced is the decline in glucose entry to the brain, and the greater is its energy deprivation. In other words, the brain is chronically energy-deprived in the event of energy excess.

Muscle proteins are degraded as a back-up supply to the energy-deprived (hungry) brain; the break-down products are transported to the liver and converted to glucose, which is released into the circulation, further increasing blood glucose concentration, and adding to the brain's energy crisis. Degraded muscle is the sign of a degraded brain. A diabetic body is a signal of a diabetic brain.

Given that high levels of glucose suppress glutamine synthetase, is there also evidence of excess glucose degrading muscle? In February 2019, a study published in the *Journal of Clinical Investigation Insight* by a group of scientists at Kobe University in Okazaki, Japan, answered the question.[8] Their results revealed that hyperglycaemia promotes muscle atrophy. Paton's work in 1903 had been beautifully confirmed, a century later.

## Fuel, fuel pump and governor: Lessons from sea sponges

Not many of us would consider the sea creatures sponges as high in the intelligence index of living organisms, but that may be unfair to that ancient and humble phylum. Indeed, it seems that we may have much to learn from these primaeval animals. It now appears that, although they may be the oldest multicellular animal in the evolution of life, with a primitive nervous system, they had already solved the problem of energy regulation some 500 million years ago – not bad for a simple animal that lacks internal organs, and which feeds mainly on bacteria and water-borne nutrients that it filters from the sea. Sponges use insulin-type signalling as their key energy-regulating mechanism. Since they have been so successful in evolutionary terms, we may conclude that this mechanism is highly efficient. There are apparently no known scientific records of obese, diabetic or demented sponges!

The wonderful system of energy regulation that has made sponges so successful – there are around 10,000 species of them in existence today after 500 million years of evolution – is exquisitely organised to achieve balance by opposing the governor (the mechanism in an engine that automatically maintains the speed/power of a process regardless of the load – insulin in all animate species) to the fuel (glucose) in an inverse and dynamic relationship – glucose regulates insulin (the governor) and insulin regulates glucose (the fuel), with the glutamatergic system providing the pump which counter-regulates the governor.

This ancient and conserved tripartite arrangement has never been equalled by any artificial energy-regulating system. Mechanical governors of all types and sophistication have been created by innovative engineers, and installed in energy-consuming engines and machines, but it is fair to say that none has equalled the efficiency of energy control in animate species over 500 million years of selective evolutionary history.

*Body energy is controlled from the brain and insulin functions as the overall fuel-governing hormone.*

For most of the last century insulin was viewed as the hormone that regulated glucose levels in the human body, and that the brain was exempt from that relationship. After a meal, and as glucose levels in the circulation increased, the pancreas responded to glucose by releasing insulin and thereby opening cells to glucose uptake, thus controlling blood glucose concentration. As glucose was cleared from the circulation, the pancreas sensed the lowered level and insulin production and release were reduced.

The mutual and reverse regulation that was the brilliant solution found by sponges 500 million years ago still exists throughout the animal kingdom. However, we now understand that insulin is intimately involved in brain energy dynamics, and that body energy is always controlled from the brain (as Claude Bernard and Noel Paton had observed), and that insulin functions as the overall fuel-governing hormone.[9] We are beginning to understand that insulin works in mutual and interdependent cooperation with the brain fuel regulator, the enzyme glutamine synthetase – insulin regulates glutamine synthetase and glutamine synthetase regulates insulin.

## How to grow and lose a brain: Lessons from sea squirts

Another ancient group of species, sea squirts, are a fascinating example of brain/body polarity and energy partition. Born as a small tadpole-like creature, they develop a brain and spinal cord after birth and navigate through the water (for which cognition is certainly required to avoid predators and ensure survival), but when they find a suitable rock or sunken ship to attach to, they digest their energy-expensive brain, which is no longer required. After attaching, the sea squirt remains stationary and simply filters nutrients and food energy from the water.[10]

These clever little animals demonstrate that bodies may precede brains, and that the brain is an additional extra organ that may improve survival potential but at a high energy cost. How does the sea squirt rid itself of its hungry and redundant brain? There appear to be no studies on this question so we have to theorise. It may be that it simply reduces energy provision, a strategy that saves energy and would result in death of brain cells, and their breakup and digestion. The body in this case rules.

In modern humans a similar chronic energy deficiency leads to a series of degenerative brain conditions that result in cognitive impairments and dementia. The body grows at the expense of the brain. The brain shrinks. The mechanism is hyperinsulinaemia suppressing the brain's fuel pump.

As we have seen, the problem for the human brain is that it secures its energy from the body. The brain has no direct access to food/energy resources. Every nanogram of glucose essential to brain function and survival must be provisioned by the body. However, this dependence is anything but passive. The brain actively pumps glucose from the bloodstream into the glia that supply neurones with energy, a mechanism that is governed by insulin and glutamine synthetase in cooperative regulatory and counter-regulatory interaction.

*The brain has no internal energy store and must get all its energy from the body but if the fuel pump is compromised the body grows and the starving brain shrinks.*

Insulin regulates glutamine synthetase, the human brain's fuel pump.[11] Glutamine synthetase counter-regulates insulin via glutamine, the product of the G/G cycle and glutamine synthetase itself. In other words, the fuel pump and governor regulate not only fuel metabolism but each other, a beautiful evolutionary survival strategy.[12]

I cannot overemphasise the importance of these two research papers that show the interrelationship of insulin and glutamine synthetase, yet the research by Ola and colleagues has been cited only twice since its publication!

## Type 2 diabetes and inflammation

As discussed in Chapter 4 (page 51), inflammation is a major influence on each of the sugar sickness syndromes via oxidation of glutamine synthetase in glia. However, inflammation as a factor in metabolic (energy dysregulation) diseases and sugar sickness syndromes has emerged only recently, and was almost unknown in the 20th century.

Aspirin (acetylsalicylic acid) is one of the most widely used drugs in the history of medicine. It was originally derived from the willow tree, which is rich in salicylates. These plants have appeared on clay tablets dating back to ancient Egypt. The formula in use today was first synthesised in 1853 by the French chemist, Charles Frederic Gerhardt. It is a pain reliever and reduces fever and inflammation.

In November 1957, a seminal paper was published in the *British Medical Journal* that shed new light on our understanding of diabetes, by a trio of researchers at the Clinical Chemotherapeutic Research Unit of the Medical Research Council, Western Infirmary, Glasgow.[13] The authors observed that rheumatic fever, a condition of immune attack on the heart and other tissues, seemed to alleviate diabetes, and they surmised that aspirin, which is used as a treatment for the condition, might have been a factor. It was previously known that salicylates improved blood glucose control. They encountered a known diabetic patient whose urine was glucose free and his blood glucose level normal, a seeming contradiction. However, he was receiving aspirin to treat his rheumatic fever. When the aspirin was withdrawn, his diabetes symptoms returned.

Aspirin is a well-recognised anti-inflammatory medication, and the questions posed by this historic study may be formulated as:

1.  Is inflammation a factor in diabetes and, if so, what might be the mechanism that determines the outcome?

2. Where might any such mechanism exert its influence – in the body or brain?
3. Might insulin also be involved?

Modern post-millennial humans express two major impairments of glucose regulation that render them susceptible to diabetes – insulin resistance and hyperinsulinaemia. A study published in 2006 in the *Journal of Clinical Investigation* established that inflammation can indeed cause insulin resistance via a variety of inflammatory pathways, including cytokines and chemokines.[14] Is it then possible that insulin resistance might affect the brain and its energy regulatory pathway?

*Aspirin reduces inflammation and it also reduces diabetes symptoms suggesting these are associated with inflammation.*

As we have seen, insulin is the key regulating hormone in brain energy uptake via the enzyme glutamine synthetase. Hyperinsulinaemia and related insulin resistance impair glutamine synthetase, an essential element in the human brain's fuel pump. Blocking glutamine synthetase in microglia (the brain's immune cells) is the key mechanism driving inflammation in the brain, and inflammatory cytokines inhibit glutamine synthetase, a vicious and toxic pathological cycle. Aspirin may therefore intervene by reducing inflammation, improving insulin sensitivity, freeing glutamine synthetase activity, improving glucose transfer into the brain, and thereby reducing blood glucose concentration. Studies are now emerging that confirm a neuroprotective role for aspirin, and show that aspirin influences the glutamatergic pathway.[15]

# How the anti-diabetic drug metformin works

*Galega officinalis* is a lovely herbaceous plant that grows in North Africa, Asia and Western Europe. The plant has been used as a herbal medicine for many centuries. In Europe it is popularly known as French lilac, and in the United Kingdom as goat's rue. In the 19th century, investigation of its potential benefits discovered two phytochemicals that contributed to glucose-lowering effects, galegine and guanidine. This led to several related compounds being formulated in the early 20th century, including what later became known as metformin. However, interest in these compounds soon waned due to the discovery of insulin, which became more widely available during the 1930s. Then in 1957, a French physician, Dr Jean Sterne, pioneered metformin as a successful treatment for type 2 diabetes. He named the compound 'glucophage', as in a 'glucose eating' molecule, from the Greek *phagein* – 'to eat'.

Glucophage has become the most widely prescribed anti-diabetic medication in history and is still routinely prescribed to patients in more than 100 countries. According to the pharmaceutical company Merck, its mechanisms of action are due to its inhibiting the formation and release of glucose from the liver, its reduction of glucose absorption in the gut and its improving insulin sensitivity, which increases glucose delivery into tissues such as muscle. Each of these actions leads to reduced blood glucose concentrations. The pivotal moment in the history of this plant-derived medicine was in 1998, when the famous UK Prospective Diabetes Study, which had followed patients newly diagnosed with type 2 diabetes over 20 years, was published in the *Lancet*.[16] The researchers discovered that intensive glucose control with metformin appeared to decrease the risk of diabetes-related endpoints in overweight diabetic patients, and was associated with less weight gain and fewer hypoglycaemic episodes than were seen with insulin and other anti-diabetic drugs.

Although there is no reason to doubt that this description of the action of glucophage/metformin is accurate, it fails to account for the wide variety of pathways that this molecule modulates, and completely avoids an understanding of a more central and upstream mechanism that would integrate the diversity of its actions. It is notable that metformin is now being trialled for its potential in Alzheimer's disease, with the prospect of improved memory and cognitive outcomes. In other words, is there a central (brain) involvement of metformin?

In September 2018, an important but overlooked study was published in the *Journal of Biomedical Science and Engineering* by a group of medical scientists in two African countries, at the Universities of Kampala in Uganda, and Ifakara in Tanzania.[17] The researchers examined the role of metformin and garlic in the brains of diabetic rats and found remarkable results. The hippocampus is a key memory and cognitive regulating area of the brain in humans and rats. Garlic extract increased the level of glutamine synthetase. Metformin *doubled* it in the hippocampus, demonstrating potent neuroprotective effects.

*Type 2 diabetes is a centrally modulated disease that impairs cognition via the suppression of the enzyme glutamine synthetase.*

This is an historic study and opens the way to a completely new understanding of the actions of metformin, but perhaps more significantly it is the first clear indication that type 2 diabetes is a centrally modulated disease that impairs cognition via impaired glutamine synthetase. The teams from Kampala and Ifakara should be congratulated for their pioneering work. No such recognition has occurred, however, in the four years since publication; the study has garnered exactly one citation. (It is noteworthy that these scientists had recapitulated the work of Claude Bernard in the 19th century who discovered the role of the brain in glucose regulation, which had been forgotten for more than a century and a half.)

Glutamine synthetase is the enzyme of cognition, communication and language, as I described in Chapters 1 and 2. Type 2 diabetes is becoming increasingly recognised as a neurodegenerative condition. The vital finding by the African researchers is a mighty step forward in our understanding of diabetes and metformin: a major influence of metformin is to be active in the glia that house the enzyme glutamine synthetase and convert toxic glutamate to benign and beneficial glutamine. Type 2 diabetes is expressed by low glucose energy metabolism in the brain. These findings point to the improved transport (pumping) of glucose from the bloodstream into the brain, thereby reducing blood glucose concentration in favour of improved brain energy status and cognition.

Pharmaceutical companies that manufacture anti-diabetic medications are invited to learn from this brilliant African study. However, this mechanism has already been 'known' for 100 million years by the honeybee, in its evolutionary co-evolution with the flowering plants (angiosperms). During flight and foraging, the honeybee carries 50 times the sugar levels of humans. Its brain and cognitive proficiencies should be overwhelmed by oxidative and inflammatory mechanisms caused by high circulating levels of sugars. But they are not. The honeybee brain and its flight muscles are beautifully protected by the bioflavonoids found in honey (see Chapter 9), the sugar police that accompany this dangerous fuel to the glia, where the glutamate/glutamine cycle occurs, and from which glucose is transferred onwards to energy-hungry neurones.

## Bariatric surgery for type 2 diabetes: What this tells us about the relationship between diabetes and obesity

Bariatric (weight loss) surgery includes a variety of gastric bypass interventions that modulate the gut so that intake of food and calories is reduced. The procedures have proved to be highly effective in reducing weight and improving health outcomes, such as cardiovascular risks but nowhere more so than for type 2 diabetes. In 1995 a team from the School of Medicine and Human Performance Laboratory at East Carolina University, USA, published a study that was profoundly informative.[18] In this historic study, the authors described bariatric surgery not simply as effective in treating type 2 diabetes, but the *most effective* treatment.

The authors were able to report that their surgical interventions in obese diabetic patients with poorly controlled blood glucose levels, restored and maintained normal levels of glucose and insulin for up to 14 years, a much higher degree of diabetic control than any other medical strategy. However, the most significant finding was that blood glucose concentrations were reduced within days of the procedure, *long before weight loss kicked in*. The weight loss was a downstream event, secondary to the lowered blood glucose concentration. This has significant implications for our understanding of the relationship between obesity and type 2 diabetes.

## In summary...

In this chapter I have shown that type 2 diabetes is essentially a brain and neurodegenerative disease caused by excess glucose energy disabling the brain's fuel pump – the enzyme glutamine synthetase.

Elliott P Joslin was the most famous American diabetic physician of the 20th century. He pioneered a dietary approach to the condition, developing a starvation diet that we would now characterise as a ketogenic diet. When insulin became available in the early 1920s, he became the leading physician in its use and was involved in diabetic education throughout his life. He developed a form of rigorous glucose control which was vindicated decades later. However, Joslin could not accept that excess consumption of refined carbohydrates and sugars was causative and believed that fats were the major influence. This predated the work of Ancel Keys who promoted the notion that fats were the major influence in cardiovascular disease. This 'double sugar blindness' has resulted in an explosion of type 2 diabetes from the late 20th century.

There is a very simple way to indicate whether excess sugars and not fats are the driving force of type 2 diabetes. We know that this condition occurs increasingly in children who are younger than 10 years of age. Do children consume excess fats/ oils in their breakfast meals, lunches, dinner and snacks? Are fats in breakfast cereals? Are childhood energy drinks loaded with oils? Are the energy bars, biscuits, confections and cookies that they love fat enriched? To pose the question is to answer it.

Excess circulating glucose damages every cell, organ and tissue in the human organism, including initially and primarily the brain. The damage occurs from conception to death, in the foetus via the maternal circulation, and postnatally via overconsumption. We may therefore identify late-modern (post 1970s) *Homo sapiens* as sugar-sick and expressing a form of chrono-diabetes.

# Chapter 7

# Sugar sickness syndrome #3: Alzheimer's disease

---

**Note on dementia**

Dementia is not a disease in itself but a group of symptoms that can have many different causes. Over 60 have been identified but the most common is Alzheimer's disease. This chapter is specifically about that condition, but some of the research quoted has looked at 'dementia' rather than any one specific cause; where that is the case I have said 'dementia' and not Alzheimer's so this is not a slip but a decision to reflect research findings as closely as possible.

---

Alois Alzheimer was born in Bavaria in 1864. As a student he studied medicine at the Universities of Berlin, Tubingen and Wurzburg. After qualifying, he became both a neuropathologist and a psychiatrist and took up the study of mental health. In 1901, he became interested in a 51-year-old patient at the Frankfurt asylum, Auguste Deter, who was showing unusual symptoms of short-term memory loss. When his patient died in 1906, he examined her brain microscopically and discovered, for the first time, amyloid plaques and neurofibrillary tangles. These anatomical findings have become synonymous with the disease that bears his name and which has accelerated dramatically in incidence since his discovery, and in particular since the 1970s.

There are currently around 50 million people diagnosed with Alzheimer's disease worldwide. It is just one cause of dementia, the loss of cognitive functioning, but it is the most common by far, with vascular dementia (due to the brain receiving insufficient oxygen) coming second. Its prevalence has been doubling every 20 years, and a new diagnosis is made every 65 seconds.[1] It has increased in a similar manner to obesity and type 2 diabetes. Furthermore, according to Alzheimer's Disease International, only one in four people with dementia have been diagnosed, and therefore the real figure is around 200 million globally.[2]

On 7 January 2022, the *Lancet* published a comprehensive report on the projected prevalence of dementia globally by 2050.[3] This was an analysis of forecasts in 195 countries and based on four important risk factors: smoking, obesity, high blood sugar and less education. The authors forecast that by 2050, 153 million people would be living with dementia worldwide. It is notable that they included among the causative factors, receiving less

*Figure 5: Trends in sugar consumption and Alzheimer's disease from 1960 to now*

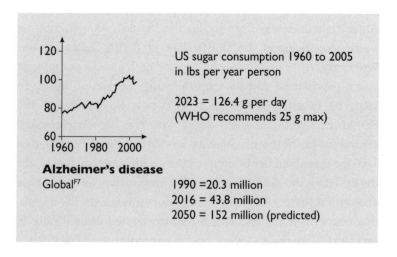

US sugar consumption 1960 to 2005 in lbs per year person

2023 = 126.4 g per day
(WHO recommends 25 g max)

**Alzheimer's disease**
Global[F7]

1990 = 20.3 million
2016 = 43.8 million
2050 = 152 million (predicted)

education. Being relatively less educated is not a metabolic disease but each of the three other factors – smoking, obesity and high blood sugar – is or causes them. Smoking is a recognised risk for type 2 diabetes; it raises blood glucose concentration in a similar fashion to air pollution (see page 72) and causes insulin resistance, impairing glucose delivery into cells and tissues. Raised blood glucose concentration oxidatively degrades the human brain's fuel pump, the enzyme glutamine synthetase, thereby depriving the brain of energy, and is the major influence on impaired cognition, communication and language – dementia.

The authors failed to note that a similar condition of impaired cognition, communication and language (the autism spectrum disorders) already exceeded Alzheimer's disease by a large margin – it currently affects around 140 million individuals and doubles in prevalence every five years. Also notable is that the authors *make no mention of fats*. According to the health institutions and a large proportion of the scientific community globally, fats are the major influence in metabolic diseases. Therefore, without being aware of the revolutionary implications of their conclusions, these authors have overthrown half a century of scientific nonsense propagated by academia, the health institutions, governments and the sugar corporations. Not that anybody noticed – this historic and revelatory study appeared briefly in the media over a few days and was quickly forgotten. The toxic influence of sugars rapidly dropped out of sight.

## What is Alzheimer's disease?

Alzheimer's disease is a progressive neurodegenerative disease characterised by declining cognition, social communication and language (dementia) plus the increasing loss of neural control of all major body functions, which is the leading cause of death in this condition. In addition, chronic reductions in energy levels, and impaired expression of hormones and neurotransmitters contribute to disorderly signalling and neurotransmission, with multiple negative effects. A 2020 study found that, from the time of diagnosis until institutionalisation was 3.9 years and until death, 5 years.[4] In post-mortem examination of the brain Alzheimer's is associated with the presence of the extracellular amyloid plaques and intracellular neurofibrillary tangles first identified by Alois Alzheimer, plus the loss of neurones and synapses combined with oxidative and inflammatory damage.

This neurological disease has devastating consequences for both the patient and their family, and places intolerable burdens on healthcare. Over time disorientation and loss of memory, cognition, communication and language increase. Eventually the brain loses control of vital organs and functions, and death follows. There are no successful treatments available, despite several decades of research. In the 1990s, the accumulation of amyloid, an extracellular protein, seemed to offer an explanation, but this is increasingly being questioned. Drugs that reduce deposition of amyloid have had no significant benefit.

Increasingly Alzheimer's disease is being diagnosed at ever younger ages. This suggests that growing older may not be the fundamental driving force and that some other environmental influence, such as diet, may be a significant factor. Studies are now implicating sugar as this generating influence. Recently, several researchers have associated Alzheimer's disease with type 2 diabetes and with insulin resistance, and they have described the condition as 'type 3 diabetes', or 'diabetes of the brain'. Both obesity and type 2 diabetes are associated with an increased risk of Alzheimer's and each of these is driven by excess consumption of sugar.

## Is Alzheimer's disease type 3 diabetes?

The evidence suggests that type 3 diabetes is an accurate name and this increases by the day. A study in 2020 by a combined team from Vietnam and Korea addressed this question,[5] and observed that the notion of type 3 diabetes offers the potential for a plethora of proactive future strategies to exert beneficial effects against cognitive impairments.

One of the defining hallmarks of cognitive decline in type 2 diabetes is that of reduced energy availability to neurones. As we have seen, this is due to suppression of the brain's fuel pump – the enzyme glutamine synthetase – by excess sugar consumption. This suppression would result in significant loss of neurones and synapses. Brain energy reduction in Alzheimer's disease would constitute a potential link to similar reductions in type 2 diabetes and such reduction has been identified.

In 2009, a significant study by a team from the Department of Psychiatry at New York School of Medicine, USA, and published in the *European Journal of Nuclear Medicine and Molecular Imaging*,[6] examined cognitively normal elderly patients, and patients with mild cognitive decline over several years, using brain scans to determine brain energy levels (cerebral metabolic rate). They found progressive reductions in cerebral metabolic rate years in advance of progression to an Alzheimer's diagnosis.

*Progressive reductions in brain metabolic rate can be detected years before Alzheimer's symptoms appear.*

This finding poses another question: Is this reduction in metabolic rate in the brain consistent with impaired glutamine synthetase activity? Such a finding would point to reduced glutamate/glutamine cycling in glia (the cells that supply the neurones with energy and nutrients), and impaired glutamine synthetase functioning, the essential enzyme required for pumping glucose/energy into the brain.

An earlier study, in April 2000, published in *Neurochemistry International*, had already addressed this very question.[7] This study by Stephen Robinson at the Department of Psychology, Monash University, Australia, may prove to be one of the key contributions to understanding the neurodegeneration of Alzheimer's disease in the 21st century. The study's most striking finding was the expression of glutamine synthetase in the *neurones* of deceased Alzheimer's brains and not of deceased control brains, which were normal. As was described in Chapter 2, glutamine synthetase is not an enzyme associated with neurones; it functions in glia (astrocytes) as the brain's fuel pump. Impairment would lead to loss of energy supply to neurones, resulting in neurone death. It seems that in the case of Alzheimer's, loss of energy supply and toxic build-up of glutamate would initiate a response in neurones to prevent accumulation of glutamate, via its conversion to benign glutamine, as a survival strategy.

In addition, the only way astrocytes can avoid increases in toxic ammonia is by converting glutamate to glutamine, which uses up free nitrogen required for ammonia synthesis, and therefore maintains ammonia at low levels. If ammonia were to increase in neurones it would have lethal consequences, leading inexorably to cell death; expression of glutamine synthetase in neurones may prevent that from occurring. It seems that Alzheimer's disease may be directly associated with suppression of glutamine synthetase and, as we have seen throughout this book, such suppression is in turn associated with excess consumption of refined carbohydrates and sugars in modern humans and consequent hyperinsulinaemia and hyperglycaemia.

Chapter 7

## The glial cell and gliosis in Alzheimer's disease

In this book I have identified glia (aka glial cells or astrocytes) as ground zero in all the sugar-driven non-transmissible neurodegenerative diseases that have exploded in numbers from the late 20th century on. Glia function as the host of the human brain's fuel pump and, since the human brain is an internal combustion engine, any malfunction of this vital energy-delivering unit serves to impair key human brain functions – cognition, communication and language. This deficiency is located upstream of all other functions in the brain, and all other malfunctions, including Alzheimer's disease, are downstream relative to that essential mechanism.

In July 2011, a seminal study was published by a team of researchers based in the Institute for Neurodegenerative Disease at Massachusetts General Hospital, USA.[8] The study examined the notion that damaged glia may play an important part, via a condition known as gliosis (fibrous proliferation of glia in injured areas of the brain), in the development of Alzheimer's disease. The authors found that gliosis links amyloid deposition to the characteristic neurofibrillary tangles. They also observed that glia are neuroprotective and that damaged glia in Alzheimer's disease are an indication that there is downstream neurodegeneration.

Earlier (page 60) we discussed the relationship between fuel (glucose), the fuel income pump (glutamine synthetase) and the fuel governor (insulin). Oxidative stress caused by excess consumption of sugars suppresses glutamine synthetase in glia, depriving the brain of energy. Insulin resistance causes the pancreas to over-produce insulin (hyperinsulinaemia). Hyperinsulinaemia adds to the problem of excess circulating glucose (hyperglycaemia) by also regulating and suppressing glutamine synthetase, and the toxic cycle repeats.

*Figure 6: The vicious cycle of excess sugar consumption and brain hunger*

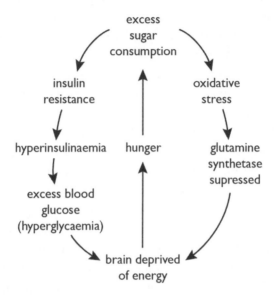

## Hyperinsulinaemia and Alzheimer's disease: A century of missed opportunity

'...It seems probable that one of the causes of hyperinsulinism is the excessive consumption of glucose-forming foods... It is possible that the hunger incident to hyperinsulinism may be a cause of overeating, and, therefore the obesity that so often precedes diabetes....' These prophetic words were written in 1924 by Seale Harris, a ground-breaking researcher in diabetes from Alabama in the USA.[9] His historic paper was published in the *Journal of the American Medical Association*, but such was the lack of interest in the relationship between carbohydrate consumption and diabetes throughout the 20th century – and continuing into the 21st - that his work has almost been forgotten, and is now only available at the University of Paris Department of Medical History.

In the above quotation, Seale Harris articulated almost 100 years ago an almost perfectly accurate account of the relationship between excess consumption of refined carbohydrates and sugars and unsated chronic hunger, followed inevitably by obesity and type 2 diabetes, and later by Alzheimer's disease. If he had added the words 'and cognitive decline as expressed in dementia', he would have fully articulated the catastrophic physiological, psychological and intellectual degeneration that is ravaging modern humanity today, such that our future as a cognitively competent species is at risk.

In October 2012, a team led by Jose Luchsinger at the Taub Institute for Research of Alzheimer's Disease and the Aging Brain in  New York, USA, published a study that beautifully confirmed Harris' work of a century earlier.[10] The authors found a strong association between hyperinsulinaemia and Alzheimer's disease, and dementia generally, and their results were supported by the finding that hyperinsulinaemia was specifically related to decline in memory over time, measured by neuropsychiatric tests.

*With excess sugar consumption, insulin production rises resulting in excess levels of insulin that have a toxic effect on body and brain.*

This study underlines a new view of all the sugar sickness syndromes that reaches back in time to the work of Seale Harris. The traditional view of increased sugar consumption was (and is) that, as blood glucose concentration rises, the pancreas is unable to produce sufficient insulin to lower glucose levels, and a state of hyperglycaemia persists, initially causing obesity and later, diabetes. However, this approach is based on a false hypothesis of reduced insulin production. This is far from the case. It seems that insulin production rises, not falls, and the resulting excess levels of insulin become a major toxic influence in the development of sugar sicknesses. This was exactly the perspective of Michael Stern at Texas University in 2012, who implicated excess insulin (and therefore excess parental sugar consumption) in autism.[11] (For more on this see Chapter 4, page 59.)

What might be the mechanisms that link hyperinsulinaemia to Alzheimer's disease? There are two critical such mechanisms:

1. Hyperinsulinaemia's suppression of the brain's glucose energy pump.
2. The effect of high levels of circulating insulin on another enzyme, insulin degrading enzyme (IDE).

## Alzheimer's disease and insulin degrading enzyme (IDE)

All structural and working proteins in the human body that are synthesised and released also have degrading enzymes that function to break them down, so that the resulting portions may be used in new synthesis, or degraded and oxidised for energy, or detoxified and excreted from the body. The enzyme that degrades insulin is known as insulin degrading enzyme (IDE), and it has been recognised and documented for many decades.

In 1994, two researchers, Ivor Kurochkin and Sataro Goto, published a significant paper in the journal *FEBS Letters* that identified for the first time that IDE had a role in degrading beta-amyloid, the toxic protein that is implicated in Alzheimer's disease.[12] This finding should have initiated a tsunami of interest in the scientific community, but did not do so, probably because the focus at the time was on low levels of insulin, not high.

## Alzheimer's disease and sensory perception disorder: How Alzheimer's disease affects the five senses

The human organism consists of two basic information systems – brain and body. These interchange energy/information internally and externally with the environment in a variety of ways. In the brain and nervous system, energy/information is largely transmitted via electrical signals and neurotransmitters. In the body energy/information is transmitted between organs via the bloodstream and the hormones it carries that couple with receptors on cell membranes. Of course, it is more complicated than that – many nutrients, such as minerals and vitamins, also function as information-processing entities.

Humans process environmental information via their five senses: sight, sound, touch, taste and smell. Information from each of the sense organs – ears, eyes, skin, tongue and nose – is transmitted to the human brain via the nervous system, and that system, including the brain, is the most energy-demanding system in the human organism. The system that transmits information to the brain from these sensory organs is known as the afferent nervous system, and the nerves are described as afferent nerves, which contain sensory neurones that relay information to the brain via the spinal cord. However, these neurones require energy to be pumped from the blood into the nervous system via the glia, in the same way that glia convey energy in the brain. In all cases, the pumping mechanism requires the enzyme glutamine synthetase, which we have seen converts toxic glutamate to glutamine via the glutamate/glutamine cycle, with each cycle transferring a glucose (energy) molecule into the nerve cell.

Excess consumption of refined sugars and carbohydrates from the 1970s on has been a major driver of Alzheimer's disease, via suppression of glutamine synthetase. Given this effect, we can expect similar deficits in the afferent nervous system and negative influence on the five senses consistent with a decline in the information pathways that humans require to process environmental information and the suppression of the glutamate/glutamine cycle.

## *Alzheimer's disease: Insight from eyesight*

As we saw in Chapter 3, the human eye has a prodigious need for energy, and any energy deficit is first expressed in the retina, the light-sensitive tissue at the back of the eye that uses three times the energy of a brain cell, and 60 times the energy of most body cells. Vision-related changes are common in Alzheimer's disease and are summarised by Ashok and colleagues (2020) who confirm that age-related macular degeneration and glaucoma are degenerative retinal conditions often associated with Alzheimer's.[13]

It is known that the toxic plaques in the brain that are characteristic of the disease can build up for two decades before diagnosis. In the near future, any individual experiencing mild cognitive decline/impairment (MCI), and who may therefore be concerned about the possibility of a future diagnosis of Alzheimer's disease, could visit their optician before their personal physician to investigate the prognosis. In September 2021, a breakthrough was made by an international team and published in the *Journal of Neurology, Neurosurgery and Psychiatry*.[14] The team used standard optical techniques to examine retinas and concluded that measurements from these retinal imaging technologies had been shown to be associated with cognitive function and impairment, and risk of Alzheimer's disease. These non-invasive optical technologies are now being used to predict increased risk of Alzheimer's disease many years before diagnosis.

Retinal blindness is one of the most common diagnoses associated with excess sugar consumption and diabetes. As we saw on page 125, Alzheimer's is being described as type 3 diabetes. PubMed, the US's National Library of Congress, lists around 1000 studies in a search for 'Alzheimer's disease and diabetes type 3'. The finding that potential loss of vision and retinal damage are emerging as diagnostic for cognitive impairment and Alzheimer's disease should not therefore come as a major surprise.

## Alzheimer's disease and sound: Insight from hearing

Sound waves travel to the inner ear where the cochlea is located. Within the cochlea, the waves agitate hair cells, known as 'stereocilia'. These hairs convert the sound waves into electrical impulses which travel to the brain via auditory afferent nerves, and are there interpreted as incoming information – the sound of speech, of a bell ringing, of a motor engine, and so on. Peripheral neuropathology, a form of neurodegeneration, is a common feature of diabetes and excess sugar consumption. Loss of hearing acuity is a feature associated with ageing, but high circulating levels of glucose also add to the injury. Risk of hearing loss in diabetes is well established.

A 2018 paper published in the *Journals of Gerontology, Series A* found, in a 25-year study, hearing loss associated with dementia.[15] The authors found an increased risk of disability and dementia for participants reporting hearing problems.

Eighteen years earlier a Swedish study had shown the importance of the G/G cycle in the auditory system. This study from the University of Uppsala, published in the journal *Acta Oto-Laryngologica*,[16] described glutamate as the most important afferent neurotransmitter in the auditory system and confirmed the role of glutamatergic transmission in the auditory pathway and the key role of glutamine synthetase in hearing.

Alzheimer's disease is a condition that results from impaired information-processing in the human organism, and the links to excess sugars and energy dysregulation via the dysfunctional glutamate system are rapidly emerging.

## *Alzheimer's disease and smell: Insight from olfaction*

In November 1944, physiologist Ancel Keys (see page 17) and a psychologist, Josef Brozek at the University of Minnesota, conducted a study of starvation and the best type of nutrition to reverse its effects. Volunteers undertook a period of semi-starvation to discover the physiological and psychological effects of prolonged dietary restriction and recovery; during this period, they would visit bakeries simply to enjoy the aroma of foods, which they would purchase and then give away. The effect of the food smells provided them with a temporary pleasure and briefly dimmed their hunger pangs. Clearly smell exerts a potent physiological and psychological effect on humans, which is translated into information in the brain.

Although the sense of smell may be less important for our species than it is for many others, for which it is an essential survival function, for our ancestors it would have played a vital part in finding safe food and avoiding dangers, such as predators and fire. Chemicals and other volatile stimuli in the atmosphere interact with olfactory neurones in the interior of the nose, and the information is relayed via olfactory nerves into the brain. This information-processing system is dependent on energy, and this is provided by cells known as olfactory glia, specialised glial cells that perform the role of supporting olfactory neurones by supplying not only energy, but also oxygen, water and nutrients from the circulation. Glutamine synthetase, the enzyme that pumps energy into the brain and nervous system, is found universally in olfactory glia.

*A dysfunctional sense of smell has been recognised in type 2 diabetes and Alzheimer's disease and is associated with compromised cognition.*

Smell dysfunction has long been recognised in diabetes.

Since the major environmental influence in the development of Alzheimer's disease from the 1970s has been associated with increased consumption of refined carbohydrates and sugars, it seems appropriate to investigate whether Alzheimer's disease is also linked to olfactory dysfunction and loss of smell.

In 2015, a team led by Professor Rosebud Roberts at the Mayo Clinic, USA, looked at this question in a study published in the *Journal of the American Medical Association Neurology*.[17] The team gathered information from 1400 adults who had the average age of 79 years. They found an association between poor smell function and memory loss, and that those with memory problems were much more likely to progress to a diagnosis of Alzheimer's disease. When followed up at 3.5 years they found 221 of those with impaired smell had developed memory problems and that, of these, 64 who had had the most serious memory deficits had developed dementia.

The connection between poor cognition and poor smell, both of which require efficient transfer of information from the nervous system into the brain that is suppressed by high circulating glucose, should concern everyone who seeks to improve lifespan and quality of life in ageing humans. Sugar-impaired processing of smell and other stimuli separates us from our surroundings and damages our survival capabilities.

### Alzheimer's disease and taste

The human tongue is covered with around 200-400 small bumps known as papillae, each containing three to five taste buds. Taste buds also occupy surface areas of the mouth and throat. They can distinguish five different flavours – sweet, bitter, sour, salt and savoury (umami), depending on the type of food and the molecular structure of its ingredients.

In February 2010, a study was published in the *Journal of Neurology* that examined the quantitative and qualitative function of taste in patients with mild cognitive impairment and Alzheimer's disease.[18] The authors concluded that there was a significant reduction in total taste scores for either side of the tongue in mild cognitively impaired and Alzheimer's patients compared with controls.

A 2016 study in the *International Journal of Cardiology* examined sweet taste disorder (a constant sweet taste in the mouth irrespective of what has been eaten) in glucose intolerance (a prediabetic disorder).[19] The authors found that this disorder was associated with diabetic retinopathy.

This is deeply significant and the importance of glutamate in the information pathway from the tongue to the brain was confirmed in July of the same year in the journal *Advances in Nutrition*.[20] This paper found that in taste buds, glutamate played a double role as a taste stimulus and a neuromodulator.

Modern excess sugar-consuming humans are losing the cognitive pathway that enabled our ancestors to find and consume the foods that provided the energy and nutrients required for survival over the period of our evolution and that may have contributed to the advance of our species.

### Alzheimer's disease and the sense of touch

Touch is a vital part of the sensory nervous system, involving specific sensory neurones and nerve pathways that transmit information to the brain. Sensory neurones respond to many types of environmental stimuli including chemical, temperature (hot/cold), electrical, radiation, humidity, light, pain and so on. They are located both externally on the skin and in internal organs and tissues. They are critically important in providing information that enables us to navigate dangers arising in a hostile environment. Pain is a major protective sensory processing pathway that provides an efficient warning signalling system for avoiding potential danger, internally and externally.

A very simple scientific method that may reveal deficits in the touch sensory information pathway is the analysis of pain thresholds – if the pain threshold is raised and pain tolerance is increased, this suggests the relevant information pathway is inhibited and action necessary for survival may not occur. Is Alzheimer's disease associated with increased pain thresholds?

A 1999 study published in the journal *Pain* found a clear-cut increase in pain tolerance was present in Alzheimer's patients, such that the more severe the cognitive impairment the higher the tolerance of pain.[21] If the cognitive pain pathway is glutamate driven and if excess sugar consumption is directly connected to high levels of glutamate, we have an important insight into Alzheimer's disease as a disease of sugar-induced cognitive information inhibition.

The cognitive pain pathway does appear to be driven by the neurotransmitter glutamate. In 2012 a review in the journal *Current Medicinal Chemistry* examined the role of glutamate in pain processing[22] and the authors noted that glutamate receptors were located in areas of the brain involved in pain sensation and that glutamate receptors were a target for new pain therapies.

*High blood glucose levels are associated with reduced sensitivity to pain.*

So, do high levels of circulating glucose alter pain thresholds? Diabetic neuropathy is a condition of nerve damage caused by chronic hyperglycaemia in which nerves in every tissue of the body, including the skin, are degraded. Although the condition may itself be painful due to degeneration of the nerves, it also disturbs the sensory pathways that relay information to the brain. Indeed, one of its key symptoms is that of numbness in the extremities, such as the feet, whereby a diabetic patient may be unaware of injury or even of developing gangrene, because the pain information is inhibited. The tactile information from feet to brain is thus impaired and *Homo sapiens,* an upright bipedal species, is losing its most important physical connection to the earth and the ability to use its legs to move from one position to another, the first major anatomical alteration since our genus left the trees.

## Of brain and bone: Do bones link early and late-life cognitive impairments?

We don't generally link Alzheimer's and autism spectrum disorders though they are both fundamentally metabolic diseases of impaired cognition and both are rapidly increasing globally. However, an unexpected and surprising degenerative connection in bones may alter that view.

Bones perform multiple functions, including most significantly, mobility, provide structural support, protect our organs, produce red and white blood cells and store minerals in the human body. They are constantly being renewed and remodelled and are infinitely complex in shape and structure, depending on their position and function in the body. They are ancient in our evolutionary history, appearing first half a billion years ago in ancient seas. Prior to this period, existing animals were soft bodied. The oldest known example of any animal exhibiting bony structure was a creature named coronacollina, a tiny (half-inch) sponge-like animal that possessed four stabilising bones or 'spicules' that seem to have anchored it to a fixed position, from which it filtered passing nutrients in the sea. Although this strategy may have been limited, it enabled coronacollina to successfully survive without high energy expenditure, an economy that suggests a kind of bony intelligence. Knowledge of where and how to fix its body to an advantageous feeding position implies cognition, however limited.

In the development of our species, *Homo sapiens,* bones have played major roles in taking us from an arboreal ape to the upright two-footed locomotive creature we are today. Our flexible wrists and opposable thumbs provided rich functional instruments for stone tool manufacture, an important step in the development of our cognitive gain of function. We may not easily consider that bones have played a critical part in our cognitive, communicative and linguistic advancement as a species, but that view has come under increasing critical scrutiny in recent scientific analyses.

## Osteocalcin and obesity

In the 1990s, a young research scientist, Gerard Karsenty, became interested in a protein called osteocalcin, which is widespread in bones. He surmised that it might be involved in bone modelling and development, and perhaps might provide hope for sufferers of osteoporosis, the degenerative disease of bone weakening that was already growing at a rapid rate in the elderly, at that time. In animal studies, he knocked out the gene that expressed osteocalcin and was disappointed to find that there was no influence on bone structure: the osteocalcin-deficient animals expressed normal bone structure.

However, he noted that the animals who were osteocalcin deficient tended to be obese and cognitively compromised. Obesity, as we saw in Chapter 5, is a breakdown of energy regulation in the body, and reduced cognition is indicative of energy deficiency in the brain. Rather than abandon his research, he continued to study osteocalcin and focused on just how this protein (acting as a hormone) could influence both energy regulation and cognition, suggesting that it might have a direct influence on the brain.

In 2015, Karsenty, who by then had become the Paul A Marks MD Professor of Genetics and Medicine at Columbia University, published a paper that reviewed his findings.[23] In this review, and a series of studies, he and co-author Wei showed that bone is a hormone-producing organ and that the hormone it secretes, osteocalcin, crosses the blood-brain barrier and affects memory and cognition, in addition to neurodevelopment. He also found that this hormone regulates energy metabolism by stimulating insulin production in the pancreas.

Human bone is a vast and energy-expensive organ. We may imagine that bone is a fixed structural material, rather like steel in modern buildings, but that is incorrect. It is in a constant dynamic state of breakdown and rebuilding, and the energy required is large. It seems that osteocalcin, although not directly involved in the promotion of bone structure, does regulate the partition (rationing) of energy that enables this process to occur.[24] If energy transport into bone is impaired, as it is in diabetes, bone mineral deposition is paradoxically increased, and not decreased, probably as a counter-response to increase strength. However, this renders bone more brittle, and therefore more vulnerable to fracture. Diabetes is a condition recognised as associated with increased risk of bone fractures.[25]

Professor Karsenty's seminal work raises another interesting question: What might be the connection between bone function and cognition?

### Energy regulation

The development of skeletal support and, a bit later, cognition appeared not far apart in evolutionary time scales (around half a billion years ago); both functions were prodigious energy consumers, and both required that the energy available would be divided (partitioned) between and delivered to the required organs efficiently and economically. Insulin (another early evolutionary influence from the same period) is the key energy-regulating hormone in both the brain and body. In the body, insulin delivers energy directly into the cells of organs and tissues. In the brain, as we have seen, insulin regulates the enzyme glutamine synthetase that pumps glucose energy from the bloodstream into the glia for onward transfer into neurones. The role of osteocalcin, therefore, in influencing insulin production and thereby energy regulation and partition, links bone with cognition, two seemingly separate functions critical to development but equally connected via energy, and therefore glucose provision, control and partition.

## Alzheimer's disease and osteoporosis

Alzheimer's disease has traditionally been regarded as a condition of ageing, and osteoporosis is also associated with increasing age, although that view is increasingly coming under scrutiny. We know that high circulating levels of glucose (hyperglycaemia) impair the function of the brain's energy pump, glutamine synthetase, thereby depriving the brain of energy, and that the impairment of glutamine synthetase inhibits the glutamate / glutamine cycle, allowing the build-up of toxic glutamate and the reduction of neuroprotective glutamine, leading to excess brain excitation and the eventual death of neurones.

If glutamate toxicity is key in cognitive decline, is there evidence of impaired glutamine production – the other side of the glutamate-glutamine 'coin' – in degenerative bone disease? Indeed there is.

Glutamine is vital to bone structure and integrity, more so than any other amino acid. Glutamine synthetase is the only enzyme in the human body that converts toxic glutamate to glutamine and, although glutamine may be absorbed from protein in foods, it is highly unstable and easily degraded in the gut so that its synthesis by glutamine synthetase is vital to human health in multiple organs and tissues. Declining levels of glutamine synthetase are a well-established finding in Alzheimer's disease as we have seen. In 2019, a study published in the journal *Stem Cells International* examined the critical role of glutamine in bone integrity and homeostasis (the balance between bone break down and regeneration required for health).[26] The authors found dysfunctional glutamine metabolism enhanced the development of degenerative bone diseases, such as osteoporosis and arthritis.

Dysfunctional glutamine metabolism is a potent biomarker of impaired glutamine synthetase function in brain and bone. Each indicates dysregulated energy metabolism, the major feature in all non-communicable degenerative diseases discussed in this book. If bone integrity and cognition are related, is there a connection that is expressed in those who are cognitively compromised and not elderly? Yes, it turns out there is – in autism spectrum disorders.

In November 2017 a study was published in the *Journal of Autism and Developmental Disorders* by a team from Harvard University entitled: 'Bone density in adolescents and young adults with autism spectrum disorders.' This is an alarming study. Autism is a disorder associated with impaired cognition, but also with problems in other organs and tissues, such as the gut (see page 147). It seems that bone structure is not immune, and that the connection to impaired cognition is not dissimilar to that in Alzheimer's disease. The authors discovered that patients with autism spectrum disorders were at increased risk for fracture, and peri-pubertal boys with autism spectrum disorders had lower bone mineral density than controls.[27]

This finding linking Alzheimer's disease with autism leads us into the next chapter where we will look at autism spectrum disorders as the fourth sugar-sickness syndrome, which I call 'sugar-sickness syndrome zero'.

# Chapter 8

# Sugar sickness syndrome #0: Autism spectrum disorders

**Note on neurodiversity**

Autism has been viewed historically as a medical condition, an approach that has opened many avenues of research and provided areas where some of the more distressing effects may potentially be modified by medications or other interventions. A new approach looking at the features of autism in terms of neurodiversity has developed which views autism spectrum disorders in a non-medical way. This view should be respected. Some persons on the autistic spectrum are high functioning and lead fruitful lives, although for the majority and their families, multiple challenges remain. If excess circulating sugars are a major influence on the development of autism spectrum disorders, those who are not profoundly cognitively challenged may hold the key to investigating why this is the case; they have been able to avoid much of the neurological and cognitive damage that has been inflicted on the majority, and this should offer a window onto the pathways that they have been enabled to modify positively. A neurodiverse approach to understanding autism and its social implications may be a fruitful way forward. However, if refined sugars are involved in altering the neurodevelopment of the brain in the foetus, this science should not be neglected.

The term 'autism' first appeared in the 1930s, when Hans Asperger at Vienna University Hospital and Leo Kanner of Johns Hopkins Hospital, USA, each used the word in relation to their own fields of research. The autism spectrum disorders are a group of neurodevelopmental disorders characterised by delayed or absent language, impaired movement skills, compromised cognitive development, hyperactivity and impulsive and inattentive behaviour. They are closely related to epilepsy and seizure disorders, poor sleeping habits, eating problems, gastrointestinal issues and mood and emotional difficulties. Diagnosis does not usually take place until age 18 months or 2 years, as a result of a child missing key developmental milestones.

This is commonly considered to be a 'heterogeneous' condition, indicating a variety of influences or causes, as I discuss next – that is, it is believed to be the result of a variable mixture of genetic and environmental factors. In this book I characterise it as a condition that is largely environmental, and show how refined sugars are a major influence during gestation/development in the womb. Genetic influences undoubtedly play a part, but I will show these are secondary to the effects of excess circulating glucose in utero. There are multiple genes (more than 100) that have been implicated. These genes are increasing in number and the more that are involved the less may the condition be described as genetic. There is no mechanism known to science whereby a coalition of genes can simultaneously influence a non-communicable disease. Something in the environment is activating these genes.

The numbers are significant. The autism spectrum disorders were reckoned to affect one in 10,000 children in 1980 and are now thought to affect two in 100 – that is, the condition has increased 200 times over a 40-year period. The incidence has doubled every five years since the 1980s, a period that coincides with increased consumption of refined sugar in the human diet, and parallels the increase in obesity, type 2 diabetes and

Alzheimer's disease that I have examined in this book. The evidence is increasingly strong that these conditions share a fundamental and catastrophic underlying influence.

*Figure 7: Trends in sugar consumption and ASD from 1960 to now*

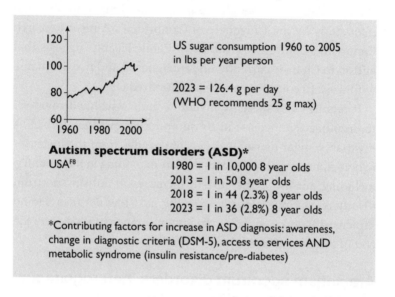

US sugar consumption 1960 to 2005 in lbs per year person

2023 = 126.4 g per day
(WHO recommends 25 g max)

**Autism spectrum disorders (ASD)***
USA[F8]
1980 = 1 in 10,000 8 year olds
2013 = 1 in 50 8 year olds
2018 = 1 in 44 (2.3%) 8 year olds
2023 = 1 in 36 (2.8%) 8 year olds

*Contributing factors for increase in ASD diagnosis: awareness, change in diagnostic criteria (DSM-5), access to services AND metabolic syndrome (insulin resistance/pre-diabetes)

Many environmental factors have been suggested – heavy metals such as lead and mercury, pesticides, herbicides, nutrient deficiencies such as iron and vitamin D, environmental pollution, epigenetic factors and so on... the list is long. The problem with such explanations is that none of them is globally applicable. These factors vary from region to region. However, there is a correlation that may be valid. As countries and regions become more developed and change to a 'western' diet, the incidence of autism increases, suggesting a dietary influence. And that dietary influence is almost invariably connected to obesity, type 2 diabetes and Alzheimer's disease.

### China and the sugar sickness epidemic

Let's take China as an example, a country that is fast adopting the western diet and experiencing the explosive growth of obesity, type 2 diabetes and Alzheimer's disease as the economy has rapidly grown and fast-food consumption has increased. What of autism? Although the figures are difficult to obtain, a pilot study by the University of Cambridge's Autism Research Centre and Cambridge Institute of Public Health suggests that autism in China is currently underdiagnosed and may be in line with western countries, at one in a hundred (1%).[1]

It requires an especially inventive and convoluted mind-set to decouple the increase in consumption of fast-food (which is invariably sugar-dense) over recent decades from the increases in non-communicable diseases that are exploding in that country, including autism. If the current increases in autism spectrum disorders continue globally over the next few decades, Homo sapiens will no longer be a cognitively competent species by the end of the current century.

## Are autism spectrum disorders 'heterogeneous' or 'chronogeneous'?

The notion of heterogeneity (multiple, varied causes) is essentially a diversion by the various health institutions and charities that are involved in autism spectrum disorders. It is a view that allows the influence of sugars to be avoided. My finding is that the concept of 'heterogeneity' should be replaced with 'chronogeneity' (time related) as the significant influence. This approach involves excess circulating glucose negatively impacting the growing brain at differing time points, and therefore expressing different effects as the new brain is formed in utero. This explains why the outcomes of the condition are varied – the differences in the condition reflect the timing, duration and degree of excess sugar damage to the developing foetus. There is ample evidence to suggest that this view is correct.

## Autism spectrum disorders and the media

Most of us have some experience of autism, via family, friends or our local community. However, few of us may directly encounter an autistic child or adult, and therefore our notions of what autism is, and how it affects individuals, are largely based on what the media makes available. This is highly skewed in favour of the savant syndrome, which was successfully and sensitively portrayed by Dustin Hoffman in the film *Rain Man*. Hoffman was deservedly praised for his work by a savant expert consulted during filming. However, autism researchers indicate that savant syndrome is not representative of the condition in general. The notion that autistic individuals are unusually good at subjects involving science, technology, engineering and maths is also common and not based on any genuine analysis. For the most part, life is difficult for individuals with autism spectrum disorders and their families, and for many the additional health problems are multiple and distressing, adding to the cognitive, communicative, social and intellectual isolation. For many affected children, a simple alteration of their routine may be a calamity and impact family life negatively. Others encounter chronic sleep deprivation and gastrointestinal problems, such as chronic bowel incontinence, that burden them and their families with additional stresses.

Although we think of autism as a largely neurological condition involving impaired cognition, communication and language, it negatively affects not only the brain, such as in epileptic seizures, and sleep disruption, but also multiple organs and pathways in the body, with its effects including motor problems, gastrointestinal malfunctions, immune dysfunction, hormone imbalances, enzyme problems, inflammation and oxidative stress. Gastrointestinal problems include diarrhoea, constipation, abdominal distension, chronic gaseousness, inflamed GI tract, gut permeability syndrome, unbalanced microbiome and digestive problems that may lead to food intolerances and nutritional deficiencies. Sensory processing disruptions occur in all five senses: vision, sound, smell, taste and touch. The non-neurological aspects rarely get a mention in the media.

## Autism spectrum disorders and excitotoxicity: Aggression

Aggression is frequently referenced as a form of emotional expression in autism spectrum disorders. Typing 'autism' and 'aggression' into the National Library of Medicine Search Engine (PubMed) throws up more than 1000 studies. Overexcitement and aggression in children is not confined to autism, and has been associated with over-consumption of refined sugars.

Parents observing their children at birthday parties often note that when they eat copious amounts of cakes and sweets, and drink high-energy sugary drinks, they become highly excited and, in some cases, may also become more aggressive. This is sometimes even referred to as a 'sugar rush'. They therefore may assume, not unreasonably, that the excess sugar entering the young brain causes the increased excitability and the possible fights and aggression. However, the increased excitability may not be due to excess sugar, but rather to a *lack of glucose entering the brain*, and the resulting volatile behaviour may be a form of brain excitement known as excitotoxicity.

*A 'sugar rush' is the result of **not enough** sugar reaching the brain plus excitotoxicity from too much glutamate.*

This is not difficult to understand. The human brain is a finely tuned internal combustion engine, and like any gasoline/

petrol engine, must be sparked or fired to ignite the motion of the cylinders. The sparking mechanism in the brain is the highly toxic amino acid glutamate, and this ignites the enzyme cycle that pumps glucose into the brain. Each ignition must be matched by balanced inhibition. However, excess glucose suppresses the inhibitory mechanism, the brain is thereby deprived of glucose/ energy and the excitotoxic incendiary principle, glutamate, builds up, causing catastrophic damage to neurones and their synapses, resulting in cell death and brain shrinkage.

In May 2018, a fascinating study published in the journal *Psychiatry and Clinical Neurosciences* examined the role of imbalanced excitatory/inhibitory transmission in autism.[2] The authors concluded that glutamate excitotoxicity is a biochemical mechanism in the condition that is likely to be due to an impairment in the glutamate/glutamine cycle. As we saw in Chapter 3, impaired glutamate/glutamine cycling is a marker of all metabolic disorders driven by excess glucose (energy dysregulation). This study under the auspices of the Ethical Committee of the Faculty of Medicine, King Saud University, Riyadh, Saudi Arabia, is of immense historical importance. Increased excitotoxicity is indicative of increased glutamate and impaired glutamine synthetase. Glutamate is highly toxic and must be converted to glutamine to avoid neurotoxic damage and death of neurones.

As I have said, aggression is frequently referenced in autistic children. In 2006, a study was published by a team at the Department of Neurology at Indiana University, USA, in the *Journal of Child Neurology* which found high levels of toxic beta-amyloid precursor protein in children with severely autistic behaviour and aggression.[3] The authors found that children with severe autism and aggression secreted beta-amyloid precursor protein at two or more times the levels of children without autism. This is an alarming finding and indicates that beta-amyloid protein may be a factor in autism as well as a feature associated with neurodegeneration in Alzheimer's disease. It is a finding that links these two neurodegenerative diseases, one at the outset of life and the other towards the end, both of which manifest episodes of aggression. The paradox in each is that the build-up of toxic and harmful principles may be linked to brain energy deprivation, and not to its increase.

## Autism and excitotoxicity: Epilepsy

On 17 November 2010, a remarkable article was published in the *New York Times* on epilepsy, not by a scientist but by Fred Vogelstein who was the father of a 9-year-old boy, Sam, who suffered from petit-mal, a type of epilepsy that in Sam's case resulted in over 100 seizures daily.[4] Sam had been experiencing episodes during which he lost consciousness for short bursts of five to 20 seconds. Anti-epilepsy drugs had failed to control his seizures, and his life had been severely restricted as a result. His father had heard about an unusual anti-epileptic diet that was being successfully used medically, known as the ketogenic diet. After taking specialist advice, the family embarked on a dramatic change in Sam's dietary regime. From consuming cookies, candies, cake, ice cream, pizza, tortilla chips, soda and macaroni, Sam switched to full-fat Greek yoghurt, coconut oil, macadamia nuts, cheese, bacon and eggs, cream and butter, such that his diet became 90% fat. His daily quota of seizures reduced from more than 100 to fewer than six. He was not cured, but his lifestyle improved to one similar to that of his peers, and he was able to participate in sports for the first time in his life.

*Before the advent of anti-epileptic drugs the benefits of low-carb/high-fat diets were known and used but all that was set aside in favour of medication.*

A ketogenic diet is a diet that is largely sugar free, and the key to understanding just how this works is that, in the absence of circulating glucose, the brain can use the small fat molecules known as ketones as an energy source. This approach was known and used in the 1920s, but it was later abandoned when anti-epilepsy drugs became available; as a result, the connection between high circulating glucose and epilepsy became largely forgotten for almost a century. This coincided with the official 'bad fat/good sugar' theory of the 1970s that has done so much to drive the sugar sickness syndromes now engulfing humanity. If the sugar link to epilepsy was obscured, so also were the links to the other energy dysregulated conditions – the sugar sickness syndromes.

In October 2019, a report in the journal *Spectrum*, which publishes science-based articles on autism spectrum disorders, indicated that autism frequently co-occurred with a long list of other conditions, but none was more closely linked than was epilepsy, and that nearly half of all autistic people had epilepsy.[5]

If the link between autism and epilepsy is an over-excited (excitotoxic) brain, and the underlying driving force is excess circulating glucose, the likely mechanism is that of elevated glutamate, the highly excitotoxic amino acid, in the human brain. This had in fact already been established as early as 1994, in a study in the journal *Neurology*.[6] The authors had concluded that excitotoxic glutamate inevitably played a part in the initiation and spread of seizures.

*Both autism spectrum disorders and epilepsy are associated with excess circulating glucose.*

Glutamate excitotoxicity, as expressed in aggression and epilepsy, links autism to excess consumption of sugars. The historic association of excess circulating glucose and epilepsy that faded from view after the discovery of anti-epilepsy drugs, such as the barbiturates, may not be regarded as a form of deliberate 'sugar blindness'; it was much more a form of scientific populism. However, the failure to examine the potential role of excess glucose in autism, and the condition's close connection to epilepsy, from the late 20th century on, most certainly falls into the category of 'sugar blindness'.

## Autism and dental problems

If autism is a condition driven by excess refined carbohydrates and sugar, we would expect that among the many compromised functions in various organs and tissues, dental health problems would be a significant issue. This is indeed the case. In 2011 an interesting paper on this subject was published in the *Journal of Applied Oral Science* by Mohamed Abdullah Jaber of the College of Dentistry, Ajman University, United Arab Emirates.[7]. He concluded that children with autism exhibited a higher prevalence of dental caries (decay) than a group of non-autistic healthy controls.

### *The findings of Weston A Price*

Weston Price was a Canadian dentist who became interested in the relationship between diet and dental health and toured the world to investigate this in 'developed' and traditional communities. When he visited the Scottish Western Isles in the 1920s, he found that dental health in the port city of Stornoway, a town that had access to mainland foods including refined flour, sugars and jams, was appalling. In communities only a few miles distant, but which lived on the traditional island diet of unrefined oats, fish and vegetables, and which had no access to these new foods, the dental health was excellent.[8] There is no debate among dental physicians about what is degrading the enamel (the hardest material in the human body) of modern children – it is bacterial invasions that flourish on the sugars that they find in the mouths of these children.

In 2009, a team of dental physicians from the School of Dentistry, University of Michigan, USA, published a paper in the *American Journal of Dentistry* outlining a new crisis in dental health.[9] The authors pointed out that in the last quarter of the 20th century dental health had improved due to the improved techniques and materials available to dental physicians, but in the decade since, that had reversed, and the problem of dental caries was increasing at an alarming rate all across the globe.

Dental health has a good record of providing indications about the health of our ancestors, due to the ability of teeth to survive many thousands of years in various differing soils and locations. Our prehistoric hunter-gatherer ancestors certainly had dental problems, but not dental caries, which is directly associated with refined carbohydrates and sugars, and which appeared more recently in historic times. Our European neighbours, the Neanderthals, who survived until around 30,000 years ago, showed little evidence of dental caries in their teeth, and according to recent research by scientists at the Senckenberg Center for Human Evolution and Palaeoenvironment, published in the journal *Quaternary International*, the Neanderthal diet was mainly meat from large mammoths and rhinoceroses (80%), with plant foods making up the other 20%.[10]

Dental caries is a condition more associated with the introduction of farming some 10,000 years ago, when grains were first cultivated and milled. The incidence of the disease spread from the Middle Ages on, when refined sugars gradually became more widely available, and more rapidly through the 19th and 20th centuries. However, although improved dental health technologies temporarily slowed the increase in the second half of the 20th century, that is now over, and a new dental health crisis is currently underway, which coincides with the global increase in sugar consumption. There is no 'sugar blindness' in the dental scientific community with respect to sugars. The link with sugar is recognised without question.

Less recognised are Weston Price's findings that a nutritionally poor western diet was also associated with more fundamental changes in dentition and jaw development. His many photographs show that within a generation, jaws and dental arches had become smaller and teeth more crowded, needing the attentions of the relatively new specialty of orthodontics. I suspect this relates to glutamate/glutamine problems but is beyond the scope of this book.[8]

## Autism and vision

If excess sugar consumption, and consequent hyperglycaemia, can degrade a tissue as hard and durable as the enamel of teeth, we may not be surprised that this food may also degrade an organ as fragile and sensitive as the human eye. Indeed, the condition of sugar-induced diabetic blindness (retinopathy) is growing rapidly as described in Chapter 3; the CDC estimates it will have tripled between 2005 and 2050. It accounts for around 80% of blind persons globally.

Vision is one of the key information pathways involved in the human mind and is critical in the theory of mind – a key concept in autistic spectrum disorders where the individual is unable to imagine themselves inside another's head or understand metaphor. Visual problems are also high in people on the autistic spectrum, as a group of scientists from the University of Brescia, Italy, working with researchers at the Department of Ophthalmology at Harvard Medical School, USA, discovered. In July 2020 they published a seminal review of the relationship between autism and impaired vision, a growing field of interest.[11] The authors pointed out that, while the incidence of autism in sighted children is between 1 and 2%, the incidence of autism in the visually impaired population may be as high as 50%. They referred to this finding as 'extraordinary', which indeed it is. They asked, but failed to find, whether the autistic behaviours of these visually impaired children might be secondary to the visual impairment, insofar as it affected their sensory processing. Although this is possible after birth, the evidence suggests that the major damage and pathology of autism occurs pre-birth, and therefore predates the various symptoms and behaviours of the autistic child after birth. Something else is at work that may link the two conditions during neurological development.

Diabetic retinopathy is a leading cause of visual impairments and blindness in children and adults after birth (up to 80% of diabetics are visually impaired), and therefore is recognised by the scientific community as an exclusively sugar-driven disease of the eye. Since the eye with its colossal metabolic rate is the most sensitive of all organs to excess sugar damage (page 53), it seems highly likely that sugar-induced damage may also occur in the foetus, during neurodevelopment.[12] It seems that in the case of autism spectrum disorders and visual impairments, the likely cause linking the conditions would be excess glucose circulating in the maternal bloodstream, a known potential teratogenic influence.

### Rubin Jure: Impaired vision and cognition in autism

Until recently, apart from a few tantalising hints in the 1960s and 70s, the relationship between visual impairment and autism spectrum disorders was largely absent from the autism-related scientific literature. However, brilliant work by the paediatric neurologist Professor Rubin Jure in Cordoba, Argentina, filled this gap.[13] Clinicians who had earlier examined autistic children had missed the fact many had visual impairments, rather focusing on behavioural questions. As reported earlier in this book, Rubin Jure found that autism was 30 times more prevalent in blind people compared with sighted people, and that up to 50% of autistic children had visual deficits. He also confirmed that this relationship was independent of intellectual ability, showing that cognition alone could not explain the connection.

Vision and cognition are two of the most important and vital gains in the evolution of complex species, most potently in Homo sapiens. Both are impaired in one condition – autism. Both are facilitated and advanced by the enzyme glutamine synthetase. They are also both facilitated by the female hormone, oestradiol, which may explain some of the gender differences with regard to diagnosis (see page 161). Both regulate energy income to the eye and brain. Both are attacked and compromised by excess glucose in the bloodstream.

## Water, energy and cognition: Vasopressin and oxytocin in autism spectrum disorders

We looked at the importance of the hormones vasopressin and oxytocin in Chapter 3, but this will bear revisiting specifically in relation to autism spectrum disorders. These two hormones are seemingly unrelated, with vasopressin modulating hydration and oxytocin modulating reproduction, but it appears they act on two of the most vital intersecting survival pathways in humans – hydration and energy.

*Vasopressin (regulating hydration) and oxytocin (regulating reproduction) contribute to key social behaviours that are negatively affected in autism spectrum disorders.*

In 2006 two researchers, Elizabeth Hammock and Larry Young at the Center for Behavioural Neuroscience at Emory University, Atlanta, Georgia, USA, published an important paper in the journal *Philosophical Transactions B*.[14] They found that vasopressin and oxytocin contributed to various social behaviours, including social recognition, communication, parental care, territorial aggression and social bonding, and that disruption of these central neurological pathways offered insight into autism. This was an outstanding contribution to our understanding of modern refined-sugar-driven water/energy stress and consequent negative influences on cognition.

Chronic water stress manifested in the contemporary habit of carrying a water bottle at all times is a relatively new phenomenon and is directly influenced by energy stress. Indeed, health advisers frequently advise people to ensure they are sufficiently hydrated. This connection was confirmed by a 2011 study published in *Diabetes Care*.[15] The authors reported that water intake was inversely and independently associated with the risk of developing hyperglycaemia. Diabetes and prediabetes are each associated with water loss and thirst.

Water is essential to life. The human adult body is composed of about 60% water by weight. A loss of as little as 2% is sufficient to cause mental confusion. The brain is the organ most vulnerable to any water deficit. Water fills and enables cells to function, regulates temperature, is required for digestion, lubricates joints, insulates internal organs, carries all nutrients to cells including oxygen and glucose energy fuel, and flushes out toxins and waste materials. Dehydration is a life-threatening condition.

As we saw earlier, water enters the human brain via two systems. When glucose is pumped into the brain by the energy pump, glutamine synthetase, water is also carried over via osmosis, to match the higher concentration in brain cells. This system balances the pressure inside and outside of the brain. The blood pressure in the tiny blood vessels that supply the brain is slightly higher than the inside (intracranial) pressure, and this ensures a highly controlled, steady flow of water, oxygen and multiple nutrients into the brain so that this organ is supplied with all the requirements to function and survive. The two systems are exquisitely counterbalanced to ensure optimal function. If too little water reaches the brain (hypoperfusion), the brain will lack both energy and oxygen, and brain cells will quickly die. Excess water entering the brain (hyperperfusion syndrome) is also highly dangerous, due to increased pressure.

Given this essential balance and that we have seen autism spectrum disorders are the result of chronic reduced brain energy metabolism due to excess sugar suppressing the brain's glucose pump, glutamine synthetase, we would expect to see reduced water flow into the brain also.

In 2018 a study published in the journal *Acta Neurobiologiae Experimentalis* by a combined team of researchers from Norway, USA, Chile, Egypt and Italy, [16] found that cerebral hypoperfusion, and insufficient blood flow in the brain, occurred in many areas of the brain in patients diagnosed with autism spectrum disorders. They also discovered that in individuals diagnosed with autism, there was a direct relationship between the index of autism pathology and the cerebral dehydration – the more autistic the individual, the greater was the water deficit in the brain.

*Autism spectrum disorders are associated with both reduced brain energy metabolism and reduced brain hydration.*

Oxytocin meanwhile increases insulin sensitivity, the critical measure that improves activity of the enzyme glutamine synthetase, the human brain's fuel pump. Conditions that are caused by excess glucose in the circulation, such as obesity and diabetes, express reduced oxytocin signalling. May we therefore conclude that these measures are connected, and that autism also falls within the remit of sugar-induced oxytocin dysregulation? A 2020 trial published in the journal *Molecular Autism* indicated that oxytocin offered long-term beneficial effects for repetitive behaviours and feelings of avoidance.[17] Overall, their findings suggested oxytocin might have therapeutic potential in autism.

Vasopressin and oxytocin modulate two of the most important homeostatic survival pathways in humans – hydration and energy homeostasis. Late-modern refined-sugar-consuming humans are chronically energy and water stressed. Each of these hormones positively influences autism, a condition of impaired cognition. We know that the glutamatergic pathway in the brain (the pathway of neurones using glutamate as a neurotransmitter) is central to cognitive facilitation and therefore also to impairment. Are these two hormones involved in influencing or being influenced by this pathway?

*The glutamatergic pathway in the brain is central to cognition. Oxytocin and vasopressin both positively affect this pathway.*

A study, published in 2007 in the *Journal of Neurochemistry* by a team at the Department of Biomedical Sciences, Iowa State University, USA, showed that vasopressin positively influenced the glutamatergic pathway via increased glutamate release in the cerebral cortex.[18]

In 2007, a study published in the *Journal of Neuroscience* by a team from the Colleges of Medicine and Pharmacy at the University of Florida, USA, found that oxytocin receptors were expressed in glutamatergic prefrontal cortical neurones that modulate social recognition.[19]

## Autism and gender

There are approximately four times as many autism diagnoses in males as in females. Autism is a condition of impaired brain development during the period of gestation. The gender differential suggests that sex hormones may play a significant part in the pathways that affect the neurodevelopment of the foetus during pregnancy. Interestingly, higher than normal levels of both androgens ('male' hormones, including testosterone) and oestrogen have been found to be associated with autism.

Professor Simon Baron-Cohen of Cambridge University's Autism Research Centre has for some years proposed that autism is a condition that expresses an 'extreme male brain', and this results from exposure to excess androgens in development. This is postulated to account for the autistic brain's tendency to recognise systematic patterns in the world, as opposed to the female-type brain that improves the ability to recognise social cues. In other words, boys are already naturally more autistic than are girls. This theory has been criticised by other autism scientists who point out that female hormones (oestrogens) in both sexes are also elevated in autism. The problem with each of these notions is that neither advances any explanation for the fact that all sex hormones are increased in autism. There is a potential explanation, and it is quite simple.

We know female sex hormones are neuroprotective during development.[20] We also know that oestrogens are protective against excess circulating glucose; they are intimately involved in regulating glucose levels by influencing pancreatic function and insulin sensitivity via protection of glutamine synthetase. An excellent 2006 study from the University of Maryland, published in the *Journal of Neuroendocrinology*, also showed that the major female hormone, oestradiol, upgraded glutamine synthetase in the hypothalamus and the hippocampus, two of the most important brain regions that are compromised in autism.[21]

It is therefore not altogether surprising that girls enjoy some degree of neurodevelopmental protection from excess glucose in the maternal circulation. This may also account for the additional oestrogens that girls produce, as a further protective measure. In some cases, girls produce extra androgens, but that is easily explained – oestrogens are produced directly from androgens, and therefore girls are obliged to produce additional androgens to secure extra oestrogen protection. The initial overproduction of androgens during the neurodevelopment of girls would account for an increase in male expression.

### What of boys?

Oestrogens play a vital role in neurodevelopment and in male sexual development. Receptors for oestrogens are found in the male sex organs.[22] Boys also overproduce oestrogens in autism, and this may be a counter response to protect against excess circulating glucose. However, this seems not to be successful and suggests that boys may express a degree of oestrogen resistance during the period of neurodevelopment, meaning they do not benefit from the extra oestrogens.[23]

## Sensory processing disorder

In my view, the evidence is that as a species we are becoming autistic as we lose our cognitive abilities at every stage of life. The condition known as 'sensory processing disorder' is postnatal but shares mechanisms and pathways with autism spectrum disorders and affects around 15% of elementary school children. It is consequently of increasing concern. Although it is most frequently associated with autism spectrum disorders, there is a growing scientific consensus that it may be a standalone condition that impairs daily functioning, including emotional, behavioural and psychological responses to environmental stimuli. If late-modern excess sugar-consuming humans are increasingly unable to integrate and encode sensory information from the environment due to impaired glutamine synthetase in the sensory pathways, the only scientific conclusion is that as a species *Homo sapiens* is becoming environmentally secluded – that is, isolated from the outside world. This would constitute a form of postnatal species-meta-autism, perhaps akin to hibernation and that has not yet been fully articulated in the research literature. If energy homeostasis is the first condition of life, the coupling of energy and environmental information is the second. The alarm bells should be ringing.

# Chapter 9

# Honey and its bioflavonoids

*'...There emerges from their bellies a drink, varying in colours, in which there is a healing for people. Indeed in that is a sign for a people who give thought...' Quran (16:69)*

Honey is the sweet, beatific food/fuel produced by the honeybee that may have initially contributed to the advanced intellectual development of our species and that can reverse the sugar-driven decline in human cognition and consciousness that we are witnessing today. However, there is a catch. We must, as a species, develop 'honey consciousness' and reject 'sugar blindness' – the wilful refusal to recognise the evidence that sugar is destroying our brains. We must give up refined carbohydrates and sugars in our food and drink, and if we want sweet flavours, replace them with honey.

Bees and the flowering plants with which they are co-dependent have been on this planet for millions of years. In 1978, Robert Thomas Bakkar, an American palaeontologist, wrote an interesting paper published in *Nature* that claimed dinosaurs had 'invented' the flowering plants (angiosperms) by both clearing the spaces previously occupied by the giant non-flowering plants (gymnosperms) and stimulating the growth and diversification of the angiosperms due to their voracious plant appetites.[1] The flowering plants coevolved with pollinating insects, a relationship remarked upon by Charles Darwin in the 19th century, whereby the flowering plants offered nectar and pollen in exchange for the reward of cross pollination.

The oldest flowering plant so far discovered was by Professor Quiang Fu, a researcher at the Nanjing Institute of Geology and Palaeontology in China, and dated to 174 million years ago, a period when the dinosaurs still dominated the earth. The oldest bee fossil, encased in amber resin, was from around 100 million years ago, and was found in a mine in Myanmar by George O Poinar Jr, an American entomologist at Oregon State University. George Poinar was famous for his extraction of DNA from insects fossilised in amber, an idea that was influential in the writing of Michael Crichton's book, and the *Jurassic Park* movies.

## Light and the origins of the honey bioflavonoids

So we know that honey and its cooperative relationship with the flowering plants is at least 100 million years old. We also know that honey contains a battery of bioflavonoids, which protect the honeybee brain from oxidation and inflammation, and are very much older than flowering plants or the honeybee. Bioflavonoids arose some 3.5 billion years ago, when the first blue-green algae appeared in the evolutionary record. Blue-green algae are among the earliest organisms to create energy from light via photosynthesis, and the organelles that performed this function were the ancestors of the green plants that today provide the energy and food of life.

Light is one of the most highly potent oxidative energy forces in nature. It is light oxidation that degrades the paint on our cars, doors and windows, and ages our skin. Blue-green algae were the first organisms to develop photosynthesis and were also the original producers of the oxygen that drove the energy of life. This doubly beneficial combination that creates life is also the combination that limits it. All living organisms eventually succumb to oxidative cell death. How was it that these ancient organisms were able to photosynthesise sugars as their energy source and yet simultaneously and paradoxically be protected from light oxidation?

Photosynthesis and bioflavonoid antioxidants were/are biological twins, and we gain from this ancient coupling every day in every dose of honey we consume, if we wish to sweeten our food and drink without refined sugars. Not only do our bodies benefit, but so do our brains. Our hunter-gatherer ancestors learned by collective rational sharing of information that honey could protect health and improve cognition. They understood that the honeybee was the source of this cognitive fuel, and they learned to harness this fuel without seriously compromising the life cycle of honeybees. Wild and later domesticated beekeeping is one of the greatest collective and shared cognitive leaps in the evolutionary history of our species.

*Our hunter-gatherer ancestors learned by collective rational sharing of information that honey could protect health and improve cognition.*

In June 2018, a revelatory study was published in the journal *Antioxidants* that examined the interconnections between light, photosynthesis, photoprotection and antioxidant networking in microalgae.[2] The results were compelling. In a diatom (a major group of microalgae) the authors were able to demonstrate that variation in light was the key regulating factor in the biosynthesis of photo-protective antioxidant molecules.

Photosynthesis and photo-protection gave birth to the honey bioflavonoids, via the later evolution of the angiosperms (flowering plants) from which the honeybee secures its antioxidant protection of the enzyme glutamine synthetase. From light energy, the ancient algae synthesised bioflavonoids which protected them from high-energy photon-induced oxidative degeneration, and additionally they protected the algae from the high-energy oxidation that they in turn synthesised by converting light energy into chemical energy in the form of sugar. Algae also contained glutamine synthetase – in these organisms this enzyme functioned as the key assimilator of nitrogen.[3] They set in motion the protective dividend that resulted in the flowering plants and pollination for nectar gain, and later culminated in the honeybee and the beatific creation of honey. Without these lovely principles the enzyme glutamine synthetase would have been eliminated from the evolution of cognition some 400 million years ago, and the cognitively advanced species Homo sapiens would not have arisen some 200,000 years ago.

## The French and api-paradoxes

In 1979 an article in the *Lancet* described the 'French paradox' whereby French people had a lower risk of cardiovascular disease despite a higher intake of saturated fats compared with the populations of other countries with a similar intake of fats.[4] This was believed to be due to the bioflavonoids contained in red wine. Later studies have confirmed that there is an inverse relationship between bioflavonoid consumption in foods such as fruit and vegetables, and heart disease. Also, studies have shown that bioflavonoids protect the liver and help avoid some of the oxidative damage induced by alcohol consumption.

If French red wine consumption offers a paradox that negates ill health via bioflavonoid intake, the honeybee qualifies as the most effective, the most brilliant, and the most potent modulator of such a paradox in the history of evolution. It carries in its circulation such a level of toxic sugars (50 times that of humans[5]) and yet somehow is enabled to protect its brain from destructive sugar oxidation, express its colossal metabolic rate, articulate its highly advanced waggle-dance communication, and perform its sophisticated selective mapping and gain of nectar and pollen reward during complex foraging.

Nature excels at paradoxes, but the api-paradox is unquestionably the most potent of these, and a paradox that demonstrates to us modern humans just how to protect our fragile brain and cognitive faculties from the combustible sugars that fuel them.

---

**Albert Einstein and the waggle dance**

On Saturday 25 April 2015, a food journalist, Rebecca Seal, writing in the *Guardian Newspaper*, stated that Albert Einstein breakfasted on eggs fried in honey.[6] There is no doubt that Einstein was interested in honeybees and is widely quoted (although without evidence) as saying that without honeybees and their contribution to plant pollination, human civilisation would perish.

On 10 May 2021, a team led by Adrian G Dyer of the Department of Physiology, Monash University, Victoria, Australia, published an interesting paper on the relationship between Einstein and honeybees in the *Journal of Comparative Physiology* that included his meeting with the Austrian physiologist, Karl Ritter von Frisch.[7]

Frisch received a Nobel Prize in 1973 for his discovery of the honeybee waggle dance, a form of linguistic communication by which honeybees shared information with other bees on the location of flower sources of nectar. He was interested in honeybee sensory perception, learning and memory, as was Einstein. Dyer et al reported that Frisch and Einstein met in April 1949, when Frisch visited Princeton University, USA, to present a lecture on honeybees. Einstein attended the lecture and the two famous men met the following day at Einstein's laboratory to continue their discussion. Dyer and colleagues also discussed a recently discovered letter of October 1949 from Einstein that addresses the work of Frisch and the notion that animal perception and navigation might lead to new innovations in physics.

---

## Bioflavonoids

Estimates of bioflavonoid numbers vary, but there are believed to be as many as 9000. Almost all plant species contain these principles. In plants they are expressed by flavonoid genes and have these essential roles:

- They provide pigments for flower colouration and pollination.
- They offer protection from ultraviolet (UV) light and from plant infections.
- They are involved in nitrogen fixation.

As already mentioned, bioflavonoids are ancient, having been present in algae that predated the plant ancestors that migrated to, and colonised, the land around 500 million years ago. This is interesting because it was around this period that the enzyme glutamine synthetase embarked on its evolutionary journey towards regulating energy homeostasis (balance) in the species Ctenophora (comb jellies), and in all later animate species, including humans. This beneficial relationship is most potently expressed in honeybees, and by the honey that fuels their cognitive and physiological functions, and which offers above all the quite sublime protection that bioflavonoids provide to this unique species.

Only quite recently have the bioflavonoids received the scientific interest that they merit. Without them there would be no evolution of the angiosperms, no evolution of the herbivores, and therefore of the carnivores, no plant pollination, no pollinating birds, bats and insects, no honeybees, and certainly no primates, including humans.

**Albert Szent Györgyi**

Albert Szent Györgyi was a Hungarian biochemist who won the Nobel Prize in Physiology and Medicine in 1937 for his isolation of vitamin C. He is also credited with the discovery of bioflavonoids. During World War II he joined the anti-Nazi Hungarian resistance, and Hitler signed an arrest warrant for his capture. He escaped, and after the war emigrated to the United States, where he continued his research. Although his isolation of vitamin C must be heralded as one of the great biochemical discoveries of the 20th century, it may ultimately be that the field of bioflavonoid research that he initiated will become recognised as his greatest contribution to human science and health.

There are more than 130,000 bioflavonoid studies listed in the National Library of Medicine (known as PubMed), almost all of which are from the 21st century. Nutraceuticals (food supplements) that select one of these flavonoids are being actively researched by pharmaceutical companies in a fruitless effort to mimic their benefits; the notion of preventing neurodegenerative conditions is beyond the current medical model which is addicted to 'treating' diseases, and not preventing them. Some 450 of these studies include honey bioflavonoids.

## How health professionals have misunderstood honey

The broad view of health professionals – physicians, nutritionists, dietitians, pharmacists and others – is that honey is a natural product, rich in sugars, with some vitamins and minerals, but not radically different from the same quantity of refined sugars in food and drinks. This view is nonsense, intellectually lazy and profoundly unscientific. There has been a tsunami of studies in the last decade which demonstrate that honey and its wonderful bioflavonoids exert multiple beneficial influences on neurological and physiological health. Most of the health institutions – medical, nutritional and dietetic associations – simply avoid referring to honey. This way they may not be challenged.

However, an article on the BBC Good Food website clearly expresses the underlying perspective, in this case by a registered nutritionist with the British Association for Nutrition and Nutritional Therapy.[8] The article was reviewed on 24 June 2019 by another qualified nutritionist who is a member of the Royal Society of Medicine and the Complementary and Natural Healthcare Council. This suggests that the view expressed is officially that of these august institutions. The article included this unscientific statement: '...It is worth remembering, however, that any nutritional benefit from consuming raw honey is negligible....'

We have news for the British Association for Nutrition and Nutritional Therapy. Your attitude to honey is the result of a curious episode in the history of this food that has resulted in a myth with respect to its metabolism and health properties that has prevented the public from fully accessing its benefits for half a century.

### Honey and the Clinton Jarvis effect

Clinton Jarvis was a country physician from Vermont who was interested in folk medicine. In 1958 he wrote a first famous and later infamous book entitled *Folk Medicine: A Vermont Doctor's Guide to Good Health*. The book remained on the New York Times bestseller list for two years and sold a million copies. Jarvis focused on the health benefits of a combination of honey and apple cider vinegar. Up to 50 diseases were said to improve, including arthritis, diabetes and high blood pressure. However, there was no real scientific evidence presented for these benefits, and in 1960 copies were seized by the FDA. From then until now, no western physician or academic would consider honey as a potential beneficial addition to nutrition and diet – this food was and is viewed as the same as refined sugars in the same quantity. This attitude mutated into a dogma, and no self-respecting health professional or academic would even consider that this view might be erroneous.

This was not the case elsewhere around the world, and from the early 2000s studies emerged that showed honey was metabolised differently to refined sugars. The Clinton Jarvis effect prevented western scientists and health professionals from an open-minded interest in these studies. It may reasonably be claimed that Clinton Jarvis was inadvertently responsible for honey false-consciousness or the nutritional avoidance of honey in favour of refined sugars.

### Evidence that counters the Clinton Jarvis effect

Honey is the product of 100 million years of coevolution between the honeybee and angiosperms, during which it has been enriched with a battery of bioflavonoids that have been beneficially selected specifically to oppose every injury that excess circulating glucose can inflict on the honeybee (and of course the human) organism. In humans these attacks result in obesity, type 2 diabetes, Alzheimer's disease and autism spectrum disorders.

Since each of these conditions begins with the upstream suppression of glutamine synthetase, and consequent neurodegeneration, I thought it would be interesting to check the research to date in PubMed on the positive influence of bioflavonoids on the human brain. I discovered that number was 7958 studies at the time of writing.

In answer to the BBC website statement that the nutritional benefits of consuming honey are 'negligible', there are some 450 studies in PubMed on the honey bioflavonoids.

If we characterise the initial and most potent injury that excess circulating glucose inflicts on the human brain, we may say with confidence that oxidation of glutamine synthetase, the enzyme of cognition, communication and language, fulfils that role. All other damage, of which there is much, occurs downstream from that event.

## The anthropology of honey

In 2011, Alyssa Crittenden at the University of Nevada, USA, published a brilliant study in the journal *Food and Foodways*.[9] She stated that the consumption of honey and bee larvae were likely to have provided significant amounts of energy for human evolution, supplementing meat and plant foods. The ability to find and exploit beehives using stone tools may have been an innovation that allowed early Homo sapiens to nutritionally out-compete other species and may have provided critical energy to fuel the 'enlarging hominin brain'.

Alyssa Crittenden is a medical, nutritional and evolutionary anthropologist, who studies the relationship between human behaviour and environment, focusing on evolution of the human diet, human ecology, nutrition transition, evolution of childhood, and maternal and infant health. She conducted much of her research over a 15-year timespan in collaboration with the Hadza of Tanzania in East Africa, one of the few remaining hunter-gatherer populations in the world.

In her wonderful study, she focused on the Late Pleistocene era, a period that extended from around 150,000 to 10,000 years ago. The foods that evolutionary scientists looked at on includ-ed mainly meats, and the various types of plant food that the Yoel Melamud team found in Israel.

(Thanks to the Yoel Melamud team, we have a wonderful window onto the diet of ancient hunter-gatherers from around 750,000 years ago at the Gesher Benot Ya'aqov site in Israel. They described in a paper published in the journal *Science* in 2004[10] that they found evidence of fire use and a wide variety of 55 plant species, sources of energy and nutrition, including nuts, fruit, seeds and root vegetables. There was evidence of both aquatic and terrestrial animal foods.)

This period also coincided with the development of sophisticated stone tools which would have improved hunting and foraging and would also have enabled early humans to reach and break into honeybee nests and secure both honey and protein-rich bee larvae. In tropical zones honey production depends on rainfall and in wet years honey production is continuous.

Sadly Alyssa Crittenden's seminal work has been largely overlooked, with a tiny number of citations in the decade that followed her paper's publication (48), but honey was the only natural energy-dense food source available to man that could fuel the expensive human brain, except during starvation.

Numerous examples of rock art that depict honey, honeybees and honey hunting during the Upper Palaeolithic period (40,000–8000 years ago), found in Spain, India, Australia and Southern Africa, are cited in the paper. These artistic presentations would surely only have been invested in if they represented a vitally important aspect of evolutionary human survival ecology. Professor Crittenden also quoted from a wide range of studies showing the vital role of honey in surviving hunter-gatherer groups around the world.

*A wide range of studies show the vital role of honey in surviving hunter-gatherer groups around the world.*

One example referenced is that of the Efe foragers of the Ituri Forest in the Democratic Republic of Congo. During the honey collecting season, the Efe rely almost entirely on honey, brood (bee larvae) and pollen. Quoting research from several sources,

Crittenden stated that the average amount of honey and brood collected per person was 3.32 kg, and the average consumed per person per day was 0.62 kg of honey (dry weight), which is 1900 calories per day; honey contributed 70% of the diet by weight and 80% of the calories.

## Honey's part in the evolution of the human brain

These figures for the Efe foragers are astonishing, and they point to the potential of this highly concentrated and metabolically controlled fuel supply for the growing brain as exactly the energy provision that, with its genetic potential (see page 176), could have been the critical evolutionary agency that promoted advanced cognition. Indeed, since there is no other food source available that might have done so (then and now), we must regard honey as the most likely driving energy source, and genetically fruitful agency of our cognitively advanced species.

I find this a far more convincing explanation of the expansion of the human brain and intelligence 200,000 years ago than others currently in favour. The most frequently quoted and popular idea is that promoted by Richard Wrangham at Harvard University, who offered a theory known as the 'cooking hypothesis'. This states that meat-eating and the discovery of controllable fire were the key.[11]

Eating meat would certainly have provided a varied and nutritionally diverse diet, but not the energy required to fuel the expanding brain. The brain burns glucose, and not protein. (Yes, it can burn ketones, but only as a survival strategy.) Also, the shortening of the gut (an evolutionary event that allowed Homo sapiens to carry around a much shorter, more efficient and adaptable gut) which occurred in this period would not have offered the additional brain energy that Wrangham claims — the gut uses proteins for fuel and not glucose,[12] and therefore no additional glucose energy would have provisioned the brain.

The cooking and meat-eating hypothesis is not tenable.

Carbohydrates, foods which release glucose into the circulation, may have played a significant part in the evolution of the large human brain. This may seem paradoxical, because it is the excessive consumption of these foods since the 1970s that has been driving the shrinking of the human brain, and the rapid decline in cognition, communication and language, characteristic of the last half century.

We tend to think that humans have become carbohydrate consumers quite recently, over the last 10,000 years, when domestic farming of grains developed. However, genetic analysis suggests that the gene that expresses the salivary enzyme amylase, which breaks down starch in the mouth and stomach, is around 600,000 years old, suggesting that our ancestors were foraging for, and eating, starchy roots and tubers much earlier in our evolution.[13] This is close to the period during which the brain expanded most rapidly in our evolutionary history. It seems that these hunter-gatherers had already developed a 'sweet tooth'. Since in modern humans, glucose is the primary fuel of the brain, and these foods provided glucose in quantity, it is possible that this alteration in diet might have exerted a significant influence in providing the fuel that accelerated the evolutionary growth of the human brain during that period.

Where, if anywhere, might our ancestors have found a readily accessible, sustainable, storable and renewable source of combustible energy that includes its own regulatory principles that could fund and genetically catalyse the exponential growth and neurodevelopment of the human brain? Alyssa Crittenden's work highlights the critical role of honey in the evolution of Homo sapiens.[9]

For the delicate brain to process the quantities of combustible fuel needed, its regulatory mechanisms would have needed to be highly sophisticated, and the fuel source rich in energy-regulating principles. The question must therefore be posed:

what was the source of concentrated and controlled energy that provisioned the growing brain, improved its function as it more recently contracted and became more efficient, and thereby enabled the development of cognition, social communication and language that we regard as uniquely human?

Any such fuel source would have to fulfil three conditions:

1.  To have been available in a densely concentrated form, accessible to our hunter-gatherer ancestors. Honey fits the bill.
2.  To have contained a cohort of glucose-regulating nutrients to avoid overwhelming the regulatory mechanisms that prevent flooding the brain with glucose. The honey bioflavonoids fit that bill.
3.  Perhaps most significantly, to have had the capacity to activate the genes that engineered the dramatic cognitive advance that resulted in our species. Can honey activate genes that enhance cognition? In an historic paper, Marsha Wheeler and Gene Robinson at the University of Illinois, USA, found that honey upgraded genes that modulate oxidation/reduction reactions that are involved in sugar and protein metabolism – a finding that confirms honey as a positive genetic influence on energy metabolism.[14]

## Honey and cognition

If honey is the critical brain fuel that helped to trigger the cognitive advance of Homo sapiens 200,000 years ago, one would expect to find evidence of a correlation between honey consumption and improved cognition.

In April 2014 a lovely study was published in the journal *Evidence-Based Complementary and Alternative Medicine* in which the authors selected 12 neuroactive bioflavonoids in honey and demonstrated neuroprotective roles in multiple neural

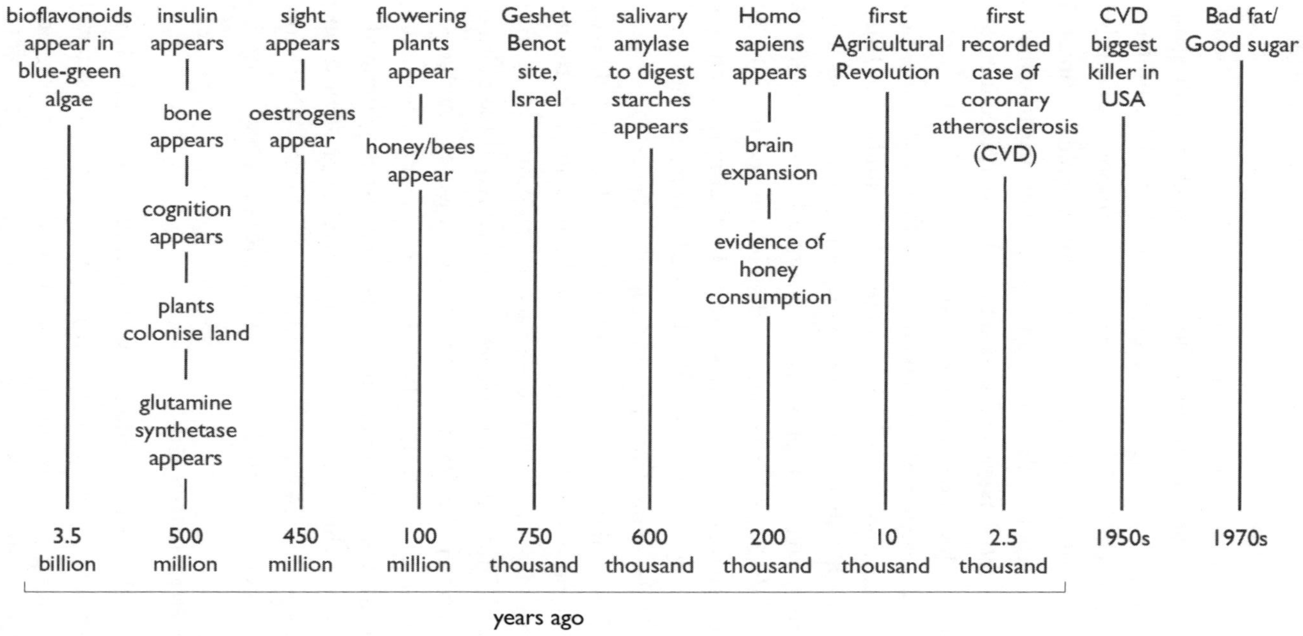

*Figure 8: Evolutionary milestones on the human cognition journey*

pathways, expressing positive impact on neurodegenerative apoptosis (controlled cell death), necrosis, synaptic plasticity and other damage to cognitive ability.[16] The selected honey bioflavonoids were: apigenin, caffeic acid, catechin, chlorogenic acid, chrysin, p-coumaric acid, ellagic acid, gallic acid, kaempferol, luteolin, myricetin and quercetin. The authors concluded that honey polyphenols (a class of bioflavonoid) countered neuroinflammation in the hippocampus, a brain structure that is involved in spatial memory, and that they also countered memory deficits and induced memory formation.

Of the 12 selected honey flavonoids in this study and their effects on neuroprotection, a momentous 7500 studies are listed in PubMed. Of course, many of these refer to bioflavonoids from other food sources, not only honey, but that is no downside. A positive study is a positive study, whether sourced from honey or fruit or vegetables or other sources. Furthermore, there are numerous other honey flavonoids that are known, and these will also add to the neuroprotective and cognitive benefits.

In addition, the honey bioflavonoids are delivered directly with the toxic sugars that they protect the human brain from – the api-paradox – a kind of sweet vaccination protecting against oxidation of glutamine synthetase, and delivered at the point of contact between the brain and circulating glucose – the blood / brain barrier. This is in the glia, where energy and information are coupled and integrated and consciousness is generated – every time we choose to sweeten our coffee, tea or other drinks and foods with honey, and not with refined sugars. What more could we ask of, or expect from, the beatific honeybee?

## Honey and nitrogen

Nitrogen is the most abundant element in the Earth's atmosphere. It is essential to life, and is found in soils, plants and water. It is the building block in our DNA and in all proteins, the molecules that are the machinery of life. Nitrogen is added to soil in agriculture to improve plant growth. The nitrogen cycle explains how nitrogen moves from the atmosphere, through plants and animate life, back into the atmosphere.

Nature excels at using toxic environmental products as essential molecules in the biology of life. In any organism that utilises these ingredients, an antagonistic supply of molecules must be provided that control these molecules, preventing excess accumulation and allowing for survival. Light energy photons are the fundamental units of cognition in animate species, including humans, but spend some time in a desert and you will soon discover just how toxic to humans light energy from the sun can be.

Oxygen and glucose are essential to life, and they are also highly toxic and therefore must be regulated with a very narrow bandwidth of levels consistent with survival. Ammonia is another although less well known. Excess levels of ammonia are inconsistent with life. It is highly toxic, and we are familiar with the caustic smell because it is widely used in cleaning material as an antibacterial and antiviral agent. Yet it provides the nitrogen that is essential to all life.

### Ammonia in body and brain

In humans, ammonia toxicity is controlled by two cycles. In the body excess ammonia is regulated by the urea cycle in the liver whereby it is converted to urea and eliminated via the kidneys in urine. In the brain there is no urea cycle, and the mechanism for controlling brain ammonia levels is via the glutamate/glutamine cycle. Each turn of the cycle adds a nitrogen atom to toxic glutamate and converts it to beneficial glutamine. This also protects the brain by preventing the increase of free nitrogen which would be used to create ammonia.

In conditions of impaired urea formation, such as liver disease, excess circulating ammonia may cross the blood/brain barrier and cause damage to glia and neurones. However, in the absence of impaired liver function, excess consumption of refined carbohydrates and sugars suppresses glutamine synthetase and thereby impairs glutamate/glutamine cycling, the only mechanism that controls ammonia levels in the brain. Excess brain ammonia is a risk factor in all the sugar-driven energy diseases – obesity, type 2 diabetes, Alzheimer's disease and autism spectrum disorders.

As I have said, the honeybee circulation carries 50 times the levels of sugars that the human circulation does, a level that might be expected to suppress glutamine synthetase and increase ammonia levels in its brain. Somehow this does not occur, and the honeybee is protected from excess levels of ammonia as are we if we consume honey. How does this happen? The answer once again is the bioflavonoids in general, and quercetin in particular.

## Quercetin, the captain of the bioflavonoid team

How does quercetin protect the honeybee brain from ammonia toxicity? The answer is already in this book if you have been paying attention, but let us look again at how energy is provided to the brain.

The glutamate/glutamine (G/G) cycle is driven and regulated by the enzyme glutamine synthetase. Glutamine synthetase converts the excitatory molecule glutamate to benign and essential glutamine, and each turn of the cycle incorporates a free nitrogen atom into glutamine, thus reducing the availability of nitrogen for formation of ammonia. The G/G cycle is the only mechanism in the human brain that controls ammonia. There is evidence that the honey bioflavonoid quercetin influences this cycle positively.

In March 2017 a seminal study was published in the Indian *Journal of Clinical Biochemistry* by a team from the Faculty of Science at Annamalai University, Tamil Nadu, India.[17] They examined the impact of quercetin on inflammatory markers in glia, in hyperammonaemic rats, and found that quercetin reduced inflammatory brain markers, and that glutamine synthetase was significantly upgraded. We know from the ground-breaking study led by Erika Palmieri at Bari University, Italy (see page 48), that suppression of glutamine synthetase in brain glia is the fundamental mechanism driving brain inflammation and consequent neuropathology, leading to loss of neurones and synapses.[18]

The researchers in Tamil Nadu brilliantly demonstrated how the honeybee can carry prodigious sugar loads in its circulation yet suffers no brain/neurological damage induced by excess sugar because of the protection afforded by quercetin, including against excess levels of ammonia that would otherwise destroy the enzyme glutamine synthetase. This study has secured exactly one citation in the four years since publication despite its great importance. Such protection of the enzyme of cognition, communication and language by quercetin is the Holy Grail of human energy regulation.

### Quercetin api-flavonoid: Treatment or prevention?

Quercetin is a plant bioflavonoid found in a wide variety of coffees, teas, fruit, vegetables, leaves, nuts and seeds. Honey is a rich source of a wide range of bioflavonoids. Although individual types may differ between honeys, quercetin seems to be present in all honey varieties.[3] The sequence of events that excess circulating glucose causes when it reaches the blood/brain barrier is:

- oxidation of glutamine synthetase, followed by
- neuroinflammation in microglia and
- ongoing glutamate toxicity
- resulting in neurodegeneration and loss of neurones – the brain shrinks.

Each of the bioflavonoids has been shown to have an impressive ability to oppose oxidation, inflammation and neurodegeneration in multiple studies, but of these, quercetin emerges as the most effective. The National Library of Medicine (PubMed) index of scientific studies lists quercetin in 5750 studies for oxidation, 1635 for inflammation and 808 for neuroprotection, raising this lovely bioflavonoid to metabolic/energy stardom.

Quercetin is not unique as a major anti-sugar bioflavonoid molecule, but it is one of the most potent, and is universally found in all honey varieties. It opposes the major injuries that refined sugars inflict on the human brain – oxidation, inflammation, insulin resistance, hyperinsulinaemia, chronic energy deprivation, hypoxia, increased ammonia, toxic glutamate and excitotoxicity, among others.

Is there evidence that it has a positive influence on any or all of the sugar sickness syndromes?

**Quercetin and obesity:** A 2016 article in the journal *Mediators of Inflammation*[19] found that quercetin had shown itself to exert strong anti-inflammatory action – a view that supports its use in fighting inflammatory disease in obesity and type 2 diabetes.

**Quercetin and type 2 diabetes:** In June 2017, a study was published in the journal *Frontiers in Pharmacology*. The researchers, who were from Universities in India, Pakistan and China, examined the potential of quercetin to improve blood glucose control in type 2 diabetes.[20] They found that it shared a similar mechanism with metformin (see page 117), highlighting it as a promising compound for the management of type 2 diabetes.

**Quercetin and Alzheimer's disease:** In 2019 a joint team from universities in Pakistan, the USA, China and Turkey published a study in the journal *Biomolecules*[21] that showed that quercetin protects neuronal cells by attenuating oxidative stress and neuroinflammation. The anti-Alzheimer's disease properties of quercetin include the inhibition of the brain changes associated with Alzheimer's disease – beta-amyloid aggregation and tau protein phosphorylation.

**Quercetin and autism spectrum disorders:** In December 2020, a team from the Hospital Infantil de Mexico Federico Gomez, in Mexico City, published a historic study in the journal *Molecules*[22] in which the authors concluded that quercetin might improve autism spectrum disorder due to its antioxidant properties.

We must be aware, however, that this impressive profile in no way suggests that quercetin in honey is any kind of *treatment* for these four energy dysregulation diseases. It simply shows us that honey, with its battery of bioflavonoid regulatory principles, including quercetin, may act as a protective brain fuel to replace refined carbohydrates and sugars in foods and drinks. Consciousness is energetically expensive and precious, and its future protection should be treated with long-term investment in controlled and regulated fuel input. Honey is that investment and the complications of excess sugar consumption that research has shown quercetin can protect against are impressive.

Each time you sweeten your tea or coffee, or food, with honey, you protect glutamine synthetase from oxidative degradation in glia, and you are enhancing your cognition, communication and language. Each time you sweeten these with refined sugars you are cooking and digesting your brain. As I said at the start of this book, the choice is yours.

# References

## Introduction

1. Erejuwa OO, Sulaiman SA, Wahab MSA. Honey – a novel antidiabetic agent. *International of Biological Sciences* 2012; 8(6): 913-934.
DOI: 10.7150/ijbs.3697. PMID: 22811614

2. Blatt J, Roces F. Haemolymph Sugar Levels in Foraging Honeybees (Apis Mellifera Carnica): Dependence on Metabolic Rate and in Vivo Measurement of Maximal Rates of Trehalose Synthesis. *Journal of Experimental Biology* 2001; 204(15): 2709-2716.
DOI: 10.1242/jeb.204.15.2709. PMID: 11533121

Note: Trehalose is a double glucose molecule used in flight by insects to rapidly release glucose to increase power output. This is a truly stunning study of flight dynamics and levels of circulating sugars in foraging honeybees. The levels of sugars in the honeybee circulation (haemolymph) may reach 50 times that of humans. This toxic sugar load in many animate species, including the honeybee, should macerate the brain into synaptic and neurological minestrone but does not do so – indicating a level of neuroprotection that humans may simply envy. If modern humans learn from the honeybee and reject refined sugars in favour of honey to fuel their brains, they may halt and reverse the excess sugar-driven neuropathology that is shrinking their brains and degrading cognition.

3. Aiello LC, Wheeler P. The Expensive Tissue Hypothesis: The Brain and the Digestive System in Human and Primate Evolution. *Current Anthropology* 1995; 36(2): 199-221.

Note: This was the first study to demonstrate that the human brain is a highly expensive organ. We now recognise that the brain is around 2% of the body by weight but consumes around 20% of the total incoming energy. We also know that energy and information are coupled, and that in humans this function is performed by the enzyme glutamine synthetase. Refined sugars oxidise and degrade glutamine synthetase and therefore compromise human cognition. As I will show in this book, honey protects the human brain from excess circulating sugars.

## Chapter 1: Sugars – the ugly, the bad and the good

1. World Health Organization. Obesity: World Health Organization Obesity and Overweight Report June 9th 2022; Diabetes: World Health Organization Report November 2022; Alzheimer's disease: Alzheimer's Research UK Report.

   Note: The Number of people with dementia globally is estimated to be 55.2 million (November 2022). Autism is officially stated to be 1% of the global population, which equates to 75 million. However, the true figure globally is now known to be 2% = 150 million, according to the Centers for Disease Control & Prevention: Data & Statistics on Autism Spectrum Disorder March, 2022.

2. Mahmoud AM. An Overview of Epigenetics in Obesity: The Role of Lifestyle and Therapeutic Interventions. *International Journal of Molecular Sciences* 2022; 23(3): 1341.
   DOI: 10.3390/ijms23031341. PMID: 35163268

3. Ling C, Bacos K, Ronn T. Epigenetics of type 2 diabetes mellitus and weight change – a tool for precision medicine? *Nature Reviews Endocrinology* 2022; 18(7): 433-448.
   DOI: 10.1038/s41574-022-00671-w

4. Nikolac M, Paska AV, Konjevod M, et al. Epigenetics of Alzheimer's Disease. *Biomolecules* 2021; 11(2): 195.
   DOI: 10.3390/biom11020195. PMID: 33573255

5. Eshraghi AA, Liu G, Kay S-IS, et al. Epigenetics and autism spectrum disorder: Is There a Correlation? *Frontiers in Cellular Neuroscience* 2018; 12: 78. DOI: 10.3389/fncel.2018.00078. PMID: 29636664

6. Einstein A. Relativity: The Special and General Theory. 1920. New York Henry Holt and Company. Translated by Robert W. Lawson, University of Sheffield, UK.

7. Lewin S. Landmark NASA Twins Study Reveals Space Travel's Effects on the Human Body. *Space.com News* 11 April 2019.

# Chapter 2: The sugar sickness syndromes – How did we get here?

1. World Health Organization. Obesity: World Health Organization Obesity and Overweight Report June 9th 2022; Diabetes: World Health Organization Report November 2022; Alzheimer's disease: Alzheimer's Research UK Report.

Note: The Number of people with dementia globally is estimated to be 55.2 million (November 2022). Autism is officially stated to be 1% of the global population, which equates to 75 million. However, the true figure globally is now known to be 2% = 150 million, according to the Centers for Disease Control & Prevention: Data & Statistics on Autism Spectrum Disorder March, 2022.

2. Sahlins M. *Stone Age Economics* Routledge, London; 2017.

Note: 'The Original Affluent Society' was a theory coined by the anthropologist Marshall Sahlins in 1966 and posed the notion that our hunter-gatherer ancestors were easily able to satisfy all their material needs with limited energy output, and although lacking extra material goods, could be described as 'affluent'. Sahlins claimed that this subsistence economy enabled these groups to lead healthier and more fulfilled lives compared to modern agricultural and industrial and populations.

3. Goren-Inbar N. Evidence of Hominin Control of Fire at Gesher Benot Ya'aqov, Israel. *Science* 2004; 304(5671): 725-727.

DOI: 10.1126/science. 1095443

Note: This study shows the wide variety of food resources and use of fire from 750,000 years ago.

4. ACC. Earliest case of coronary artery disease found in Egyptian Princess. www.acc.org/about-acc/press-releases/2011/04/05/16/22/mummies 5 April 2011 (accessed 9 February 2023)

5. Dalen JE, Alpert JS, Goldberg RJ, Weinstein RS. The epidemic of the 20th century: coronary heart disease. *Am J Med* 2014; 127(9): 807-812. DOI: 10.1016/j.amjmed.2014.04.015

6. Keys A, Menotti A, Blackburn H, et al. The seven countries study: 2,289 deaths in 15 years. *Preventive Medicine* 1984; 13(2): 141-154. DOI: 10.1016/0091-7435(84)90047-1. PMID: 6739443

Note: Keys' famous study focused on saturated fats as the key influence on heart disease. This study was critical in opposing (and marginalising) the work of John Yudkin, who promoted the notion that refined sugars were the major influence. Yudkin's work is now beginning to be recognised after many decades.

7. Yudkin J. *Pure, White and Deadly* New York, 1972. Reissued in 2012 by Penguin Books, London.

Note: Yudkin's work has been championed by Robert Lustig, a leading academic opponent of refined sugars, but after a minor wave of media interest that followed its latest publication, the role of refined sugars in the metabolic degradation of human health and cognition continues relentlessly.

8. Stephen AM, Sieber GM. Trends in individual fat consumption in the UK 1900-1985. *Br J Nutr* 1994; 71(5): 775-788. DOI: 10.1079/bjn19940183

9. Grasgruber P, Cacek J, Hrazdira E, Hrebickova S, Sebera M. Global Correlates of Cardiovascular risk: A Comparison of 158 Countries. *Nutrients* 2018; 10(4): 411. DOI: 10.3390/nu10040411. PMID: 29587470

Note: The truth is finally out after half a century of obscurantism. These authors discovered that, regardless of the statistical method used, the trends identify high carbohydrate consumption as the dietary factor most consistently associated with the risk of cardiovascular disease. This was the first study to compare the complete global statistics for cardiovascular disease prevalence with nutrition statistics from the FAOSTAT database. The authors identified areas where the data was incomplete or likely to be inaccurate but still drew the conclusion: 'we can say that in all the statistical comparisons that have been made, the indicators of CVDs always show the most consistent association with high carbohydrate consumption, especially in the form of high-glycaemic cereals, in particular wheat. Other suspect variables are alcohol (mainly in its distilled form) and sunflower oil, but their roles are limited to Europe where their consumption rates are sufficiently high.'

10. Stephen AM, Sieber GM. Trends in individual fat consumption in the UK 1900-1985. *Br J Nutr* 1994; 71(5): 775-788. DOI: 10.1079/bjn19940183

    Note: Recent stats have muddied the waters with increased plant oil consumption – so-called 'healthy' fats but many of these are pro-inflammatory omega-6 oils that have been turned into trans fat by food processing.

11. Shahbandeh M. Total sugar consumption worldwide from 2010/2011 to 2021/2022. *Statista* 13 June 2022. www.statista.com/statistics/249681/total-consumption-of-sugar-worldwide/ (accessed 9 March 2023)

12. Kearns CE, Schmidt LA, Glantz SA. Sugar Industry and Coronary Heart Disease Research. A Historical Analysis of Internal Industry Documents. *Journal of the American Medical Association Internal Medicine* 2016. 176(11): 1680-1685. DOI: 10.1001/jamainternmed.2016;5394

13. Kearns CE, Schmidt LA, Glantz SA. Sugar Industry and Coronary Heart Disease Research. A Historical Analysis of Internal Industry Documents. *Journal of the American Medical Association*

*Internal Medicine* 2016; 176(11): 1680-1685.
DOI: 10.1001/jamainternmed.2016.5394

14. Gibas MK, Gibas KJ. Induced and controlled dietary ketosis as a regulator of obesity and metabolic syndrome pathologies. *Journal Diabetes & Metabolic Syndrome: Clinical Research and Reviews* 2017; 11(suppl 1): S385-S390. PMID 28433617 DOI: 10.1016/j.dsx.2017.03.022.

15. Aaron DG, Siegal MB. Sponsorship of National Health Organizations by Two Major Soda Companies. *American Journal of Preventive Medicine* 2017; 52(1): 20-30. DOI: 10.1016/j.amepri.2016.08.010. PMID: 27745783

16. Oxfam: EU Sugar subsidies Starve the Poor. Report in Deutsche Welle (DW) Germany's International Broadcaster 14/04/2004. www.dw.com/en/oxfam-eu-sugar-subsidies-starve-the-poor/a-1169244

17. Lustig RH. *Metabolical: The Lure and the Lies of Processed Food, Nutrition, and Modern Medicine.* Hodder & Stoughton, London: 2021.

18. Hamed NO, Al-Ayadhi L, Osman MA, et al. Understanding the roles of glutamine synthetase, glutaminase, and glutamate decarboxylase autoantibodies in imbalanced excitatory/ inhibitory neurotransmission as etiological mechanisms of autism. *Journal of Psychiatry and Clinical Neurosciences* 2018; 72(5): 361-373. DOI: 10.1111/pcn.12639. PMID: 29356297

Note: Impaired glutamate/glutamine cycling is a marker of all excess-sugar-driven metabolic (energy dysregulation) diseases. This study under the auspices of the Ethical Committee of the Faculty of Medicine, King Saud University, Riyadh, Saudi Arabia, is of immense importance. Increased excitotoxicity is indicative of increased glutamate and impaired glutamine synthetase. Glutamate is highly toxic and must be converted to glutamine to avoid neurotoxic damage and death of neurones. Presumably because this study was conducted in the Middle East, it has received only two citations globally.

19. Kanimozhi S, Subramanian P, Shanmugapriya S, Sathishkumar S. Role of bioflavonoid quercetin on Expression of Urea Cycle Enzymes, Astrocytic and Inflammatory Markers in Hyperammonaemia Rats. *Indian Journal of Clinical Biochemistry* 2017; 32(1): 68-73. DOI: 10.1007/s12291-016-0575-8. PMID: 28149015

Note: This brilliant study from Annamalai University, Tamil Nadu, India, demonstrated anti-ammonia benefits of quercetin; the mechanism may be due to increased glutamine synthetase, the only enzyme in the human brain that controls ammonia levels. The authors noted that treatment with quercetin significantly enhanced the expression of glutamine synthetase. This historic study has secured only one citation in the PubMed library – a shocking indictment of western science.

20. Erejuwa OO, Sulaiman SA, Wahab MSA. Honey – a novel antidiabetic agent. *International of Biological Sciences* 2012; 8(6): 913-934. DOI: 10.7150/ijbs.3697. PMID: 22811614

Note: This historic study presented conclusions that were potentially explosive, reversing half a century of nonsense emanating from western health institutions, professions and academia. In the decade since, it has gained only 34 citations in PubMed, of which only six have been from the western cannon – that is approximately 3.5 per annum. If the study had been nonsense, there would have been a tsunami of citations pointing out its flaws, and essentially closing the door on future investigations into the benefits of honey. No such tsunami occurred; only silence.

## Chapter 3: Glutamine synthetase – the engine of cognition, communication and language

1. Diamond MC, Scheibel AB, Murphy GM, Harvey T. On the brain of a scientist: Albert Einstein. *Experimental Neurology* 1985; 88(1): 198-204 DOI: 10.10.1016/0014-4886(85)90123-2 PMID: 3979509

Note: This study showed that Albert Einstein's brain had a

higher-than-normal number of glia relative to neurones. Glia are the cells that house the enzyme glutamine synthetase – the human brain's fuel pump. Therefore, Einstein's brain may have had a higher energy processing capacity.

2. Montanari M, Martella G, Bonsi P, Meringolo M. Autism Spectrum Disorder: Focus on Glutamatergic Neurotransmission. *International Journal of Molecular Sciences* 2022; 23(7): 3861. DOI: 10.3390/ijms23073861. PMID: 35409220

Note: The authors focus on the glutamatergic system involvement in neurodevelopment including synaptogenesis, synaptic plasticity, axon and dendrite formation and cellular migration, critical to structure and function of the new brain.

3. Maltais-Payette I, Boulet M-M, Prehn C, et al. Circulating glutamate concentration as a biomarker of visceral obesity and associated metabolic alterations. *Nutrition & Metabolism* 2018; 15: Article number 78. DOI: 10.1186/s12986-018-0316-5

4. Liu X, Zheng Y, Guasch-Ferre M, et al. High plasma glutamate and low glutamine-to-glutamate ratio are associated with type 2 diabetes: Case-cohort study within the PREDIMED trial. *Nutrition, Metabolism & Cardiovascular Diseases* 2019; 29(10): 1040-1049. DOI: 10.1016/j.numecd.2019.06.005. PMID: 31377179

5. Wang R, Reddy PH. Role of glutamate and NMDA receptors in Alzheimer's disease. *Journal of Alzheimer's Disease* 2017; 57(4): 1041-1048. DOI: 10.3233/JAD-160763. PMID: 27662322

6. Rojas DC. The role of glutamate and its receptors in autism and the use of glutamate receptor antagonists in treatment. *Journal of Neural Transmission (Vienna)* 2014; 121(8): 891-905. DOI: 10.1007/s00702-014-1216-0. PMID: 24752754

7. Matsuyama T, Yoshinaga SK, Shibue K, Mak TW. Comorbidity-associated glutamine deficiency is a predisposition to severe COVID-19. *Cell Death & Differentiation* 2021; 28(12): 3199-3213. DOI: 10.1038/s41418-021-00892-y. PMID: 34663907

8. Miller SL. A Production of Amino Acids under Possible Primitive

# References

Earth Conditions. *Science* 1953; 117(3046): 528-529.
DOI: 10.1126/science.117.3046.528. PMID: 13056598

Note: Introduction of Stanley Lloyd Miller's revolutionary
experiment on the formation of amino acids on Earth.

9. Kumada Y, Benson DR, Hillermann D, et al. Evolution of the
glutamine synthetase gene, one of the oldest existing and
functioning genes. *Proceedings of the National Academy of Sciences
USA* 1993; 90(7): 3009-3013.
DOI: 10.1073/pnas.90.7.3009. PMID: 8096645

10. Seiler N. Is ammonia a pathogenic factor in Alzheimer's disease?
*Neurochemical Research* 1993; 18(3): 235-245.
DOI: 10.1007/BF00969079. PMID: 8479596

11. Shavkuta GV, Shnyukova TV, Kolesnikova ES, et al. Increased
ammonia levels and its association with visceral obesity and
insulin resistance. *Experimental & Clinical Gastroenterology* 2019; 9.
DOI: 10.31146/1682-8658-ecg-169-9-75-79

12. Gunanithi K, Dasan A, Sheriff A. Hyperammonaemia in
Uncontrolled Type 2 Diabetes Mellitus. *IOSR Journal of Dental and
Medical Sciences* 2016; 16(10): 14-19.
DOI: 10.9790/0853-1510031419

13. Adlimoghaddam A, Sabbir MG, Albensi BC. Ammonia as a
Potential Neurotoxic Factor in Alzheimer's Disease. *Frontiers in
Molecular Neuroscience* 2016; 9: 57.
DOI: 10.3389/fnmol.2016.00057. PMID: 27551259

14. Saleem TH, Shehata GA, Toghan R, et al. Assessments of
Amino Acids, Ammonia and Oxidative Stress Among
Cohort of Egyptian Autistic Children: Correlations with
Electroencephalogram and Disease Severity. *Neuropsychiatric
Disease and Treatment* 2010; 16: 11-24
DOI: 10.2147/NDT.S233105. PMID: 32021185

15. Spodenkiewicz M, Diez-Fernandez C, Rufenacht V, et al.
Minireview on Glutamine Synthetase Deficiency, an Ultra-Rare
Inborn Error of Amino Acid Biosynthesis. *Biology (Basel)* 2016;

5(4): 40. DOI: 10.3390/biology5040040. PMID: 27775558

Note: This study should sound the alarm worldwide. Glutamine synthetase deficiency expressed severe epileptic encephalopathy (a hallmark of autism), glutamine deficiency (a hallmark of excess sugar consumption) and chronic hyper-ammonia (a hallmark of all refined sugar-related conditions – obesity, diabetes type 2 and Alzheimer's disease). Clearly congenital deficiency of this vital enzyme is more potent than that induced by diet, but the indications are significant.

# Chapter 4: Oxidising glutamine synthetase, the enzyme of human cognition

1. Rzechorzek NM, Thrippleton MJ, Chappell FM, et al. A daily temperature rhythm in the human brain predicts survival after brain injury. *Brain* 2022; 145(6): 2031-2048.
   DOI: 10.1093/brain/awab466. PMID: 35691613

   Note: The authors found an astonishing variation in brain temperature – from 32.6°C to 42.3°C, a 10-degree differential. They concluded that daily rhythmic temperature variation as opposed to absolute brain temperature was the key marker of neuropathology.

2. Fernandez-Montoya L, Avendano C, Negredo P. The Glutamatergic system in Primary Somatosensory Neurones and Its Involvement in Sensory Input-Dependent Plasticity. *International Journal of Molecular Science* 2017; 19(1): 69.
   DOI: 10.3390/ijms19010069. PMID: 29280965

3. Palmieri EM, Menga A, Lebrun A, et al. Blockade of Glutamine Synthetase Inflammatory Response in Microglial Cells. *Antioxidant & Redox Signaling* 2017; 26(8): 351-363.
   DOI: 10.1089/ars.2016.6715. PMID: 2778118

4. Asmat U, Abad K, Ismail K. Diabetes mellitus and oxidative stress – A concise review. *Saudi Pharmaceutical Journal* 2016; 24(5): 547-553.
   DOI: 10.1016/j.jsps.2015.03.013. PMID: 27752226

# References

5. Gella A, Durany N. Oxidative stress in Alzheimer's disease. *Cell Adhesion & Migration* 2009; 3(1): 88-93.
DOI: 10.4161/cam.3.1.7402. PMID: 19372765

6. Pangrazzi L, Balasco L, Bozzi Y. Oxidative Stress and Immune System Dysfunction in Autism Spectrum Disorders. *International Journal of Molecular Sciences* 2020; 21(9): 3293.
DOI: 10.3390/ijms21093293. PMID: 32384730

7. Vopson MM. Experimental protocol for testing the mass-energy-information equivalence principle. *AIP Advances* 2022; 12: 035311.
DOI: 10.1063/5.0087175

8. Ellulu MS, Patimah I, Khaza'ai H, et al. Obesity and inflammation: the linking mechanism and the complication. *Archives of Medical Science* 2017; 13(4): 851-863.
DOI: 10.5114/aoms.2016.58928. PMID: 2871154

9. Tsalamandris S, Antonopoulos AS, Oikonomou E, et al. The Role of Inflammation in Diabetes: Current Concepts and Future Perspectives. *European Cardiology Review* 2019; 14(1): 50-59.
DOI: 10.15420/ecr.2018.33.1. PMID: 31131037

10. Kinney JW, Bemiller SM, Murtishaw AS, et al. Inflammation as a central mechanism in Alzheimer's disease. *Alzheimer's & Dementia: Translational Research & Clinical Interventions* 2018; 4: 575-590. DOI: 10.1016/j.trci.2018.06.014. PMID: 30406177

11. Siniscalco D, Schultz S, Brigida AL, Antonucci N. Inflammation and Neuro-Immune Dysregulations in Autism Spectrum Disorders. *Pharmaceuticals (Basel)* 2018; 11(2): 56.
DOI: 10.3390/ph11020056. PMID: 29867038

12. Cope EC, LaMarca EA, Monari PK, et al. Microglia Play an Active Role in Obesity-Associated Cognitive Decline. *Journal of Neuroscience* 2018; 38(41): 8889-8904.
DOI: 10.1523/JNEUROSCI.0789-18.2018. PMID: 30201764

13. Kinuthia UN, Wolf A, Langmann T. Microglia and Inflammatory Responses in Diabetic Retinopathy. *Frontiers in Immunology* 2020: 11: 564077. DOI: 10.3389/fimmu.2020.564077. PMID 33240260

14. Hansen DV, Hanson JE, Sheng M. Microglia in Alzheimer's disease. *Journal of Cell Biology* 2018; 217(2): 459-472. DOI: 10.1083/jcb.201709069. PMID: 29196480

15. Rodriguez JI, Kern JK. Evidence of microglial activation in autism and its possible role in brain underconnectivity. *Neuron Glia Biology* 2011; 7(2-4): 205-213. DOI: 10.1017/S1740925X12000142. PMID: 22874006

16. Fernandez-Montoya L, Avendano C, Negredo P. The Glutamatergic system in Primary Somatosensory Neurons and Its Involvement in Sensory Input – Dependent Plasticity. *International Journal of Molecular Science* 2017; 19(1): 69. DOI: 10.3390/ijms19010069. PMID: 29280965

17. Denton M. The Inverted Retina: Maladaptation or Pre-adaptation. *Origins & Design* 1999; 19(2): 37. www.arn.org/docs/odesign/od192/invertedretina192.htm

    Note: Michael Denton showed that the mammalian photoreceptor could generate an electrical response to a single photon of light energy and was capable of catalysing a cascade that massively amplified this initial signal. The amplification required vast energy input such that photoreceptor cells expressed one of the highest known metabolic rates in nature at three times that of the brain's cerebral cortex. Any decrease in energy supply (caused by, for instance, oxidation of glutamine synthetase) would have devastating results. This is easily indexed by the colossal rate of retinopathic blindness in type 2 diabetes, a disease which is one of the leading causes of blindness worldwide.

18. Parker A. *In the Blink of an Eye*. Perseus Publishing, 2003.

    Note: Andrew Parker advanced a theory as to what caused the Cambrian explosion when multiple animal species arose in a tiny moment of evolutionary history – 25 million years – and answered the question: vision.

19. Jure R. Seeing connections between autism and blindness. *Journal Spectrum* 12 November 2019.

# References

Note: This fascinating article by Rubin Jure explored the remarkable connection between autism and visual impairments. He pointed out that, to the seasoned eye, the similarities between blindism (unusual and/or repetitive behaviours in the blind population) and autism were striking. They included atypical communication, language and social skills, as well as stereotypies, resistance to change, severe anxiety and high pain tolerance. Since visual advance is among the earliest evolutionary gains of function along with cognition; overconsumption of refined sugars that deprive both the brain and retina of energy via suppression of the fuel pump glutamine synthetase is driving this loss of function is an early indicator of sugar-induced pathology in the brain and the eye.

20. Kaiser E, Galvis VC, Armbruster U. Efficient photosynthesis in dynamic light environments: a chloroplast's perspective. *Biochemical Journal* 2019; 476(19): 2725-2741. DOI: 10.1042/BCJ20190134. PMID: 31654058

21. Das A. Diabetic Retinopathy: Battling the Global Epidemic. *Investigative Ophthalmology & Visual Science* 2016; 57: 6669-6682. DOI: 10.1167/iovs.16-21031

22. Yu WS, Acquill L, Wong KH, et al. Transcorneal electrical stimulation enhances cognitive functions in aged and 5XFAD mouse models. *Annals of the New York Academy of Sciences* 2022; 1515(1): 249-265. DOI: 10.1111/nyas.14850. PMID: 35751874

23. Chung CW, Stephens AD, Konno T, et al. Intracellular Aβ42 Aggregation Leads to Cellular Thermogenesis. *Journal of the American Chemical Society* 2022; 144(22): 10034-10041. DOI: 10.1021/jacs.2c03599. PMID: 35616634

24. Lozano AM, Fosdick L, Chakravarty MM, et al. A Phase 11 Study of Fornix Deep Brain Stimulation in Mild Alzheimer's Disease. *Journal of Alzheimer's Disease* 2016; 54(2): 777-787. DOI: 103233/JAD-160017. PMID: 27567810

25. Formolo DA, Gaspar JM, Melo HM, et al. Deep Brain Stimulation and Obesity: A Review and Future Directions. *Frontiers in*

*Neuroscience* 2019; 13: 323 DOI: 10.3389/fnins.2019.00323.
PMID: 31057350

26. Diepenbroek C, van der Plasse G, Eggels L, et al. Alterations in blood glucose and plasma glucagon concentrations during deep brain stimulation in the shell region of the nucleus accumbens in rats. *Frontiers in Neuroscience* 2013; 7: 226.
DOI: 10.3389/fnins.2013.00226. PMID: 24339800

27. Luo Y, Sun Y, Tian X, et al. Deep Brain Stimulation for Alzheimer's Disease: Stimulation Parameters and Potential Mechanisms of Action. *Frontiers in Aging Neuroscience* 2021; 13: 619543.
DOI: 10.3389/fnagi.2021.619543. PMID: 33776742

28. Sinha S, McGovern RA, Sheth SA. Deep brain stimulation for severe autism: from pathophysiology to procedure. *Neurosurgical Focus* 2015; 38(6): E3.
DOI: 10.3171/2015.3.FOCUS1548. PMID: 26030703

29. Kahn BB, Flier JS. Obesity and Insulin Resistance. *Journal of Clinical Investigation* 2000; 106(4): 473-481. DOI: 10.1172/JCI10842

30. Taylor R. Insulin Resistance and Type 2 Diabetes. *Diabetes* 2012; 61(4): 778-779. DOI: 10.2337/db12-0073

31. Luchsinger JA, Tang M-X, Shea S, Mayeux R. Hyperinsulinemia and risk of Alzheimer's disease. *Neurology* 2004; 63(7): 1187-1192.
DOI: 10.1212/01.wnl.0000140292.04932.87. PMID: 15477536

32. Stern M. Insulin signaling and autism. *Frontiers in Endocrinology* 2011; 2: 54. DOI: 10.3389/fendo.2011.00054. PMID: 22649376

33. Kahn BB, Flier JS. Obesity and Insulin Resistance. *Journal of Clinical Investigation* 2000; 106(4): 473-481. DOI: 10.1172/JCI10842

Note: The authors found that insulin resistance and hyperinsulinaemia, in addition to being caused by obesity, can contribute to its development. Insulin resistance and hyperinsulinaemia are normally associated with type 2 diabetes. This study beautifully confirms that these two ailments are essentially similar excess sugar driven conditions. Yes, fats can influence insulin resistance and consequent hyperinsulinaemia, but this is driven by high levels of circulating sugars as the initiating event.

34. Stern M. Insulin signalling and autism. *Frontiers in Endocrinology* 2011; 2: 54. DOI: 10.3389/fendo.2011.00054. PMID: 22649376

Note: An historic study of global importance from Michael Stern at Texas University. Dr Stern drew from gestational diabetes and high energy pathways and foetal hyperinsulinaemia to implicate insulin signalling in autism, the first study to identify the connection with refined sugars. This study should have caused a worldwide storm of interest in the autism scientific community but did not – there have been only eight citations in a decade and only two from autistic studies, both from China. This pathway is overactivated in obesity, type 2 diabetes and Alzheimer's disease, strongly suggesting a shared excess refined sugar pathology.

35. National Institute of Aging. Exendin-4: From lizard to laboratory and beyond. 11 July 2012. www.nia.nih.gov/news/exendin-4-lizard-laboratory-and-beyond (accessed 11 March 2023)

Note: This report showed that Gilatide, derived from Exendin-4, dramatically heightened memory in a study with mice and that Gilatide is likely to be researched further to provide help to Alzheimer's patients.

36. Sandoval D, Sisley SR. Brain GLP-1 and insulin Sensitivity. *Molecular and Cellular Endocrinology* 2015; 418: 27-32. DOI: 10.1016/j.mce.2015.02.017. PMID: 25724479

Note: Insulin sensitivity in the brain is a major influence on the glutamate/glutamine (G/G) cycle. Excess insulin suppresses glutamine synthetase, the upstream problem for regulating appetite. Improved insulin sensitivity protects glutamine synthetase and reduces appetite.

37. Ola MS, Hosoya K-I, LaNoue KF. Influence of insulin on glutamine synthetase in Muller glial cells of the retina. *Metabolic Brain Disease* 2011; 26(3): 195-202. DOI: 10.1007/s11011-011-9245-202. PMID: 21626103

Note: This deeply important study demonstrates insulin regulation of glutamine synthetase. Modern refined carbs and sugar-consuming humans are insulin resistant and in the brain this is devastating – in microglia an inflammatory cascade causes cannibalisation of neurones and other brain cells, a cognitive catastrophe.

38. Cheke LG, Simons JS, Clayton NS. Higher body mass index is associated with episodic memory deficits in young adults. *Quarterly Journal of Experimental Psychology* 2016; 69(11): 2305-2316. DOI: 10.1080/17470218.2015.1099163. PMID: 26447832

Note: This is an important study linking obesity to memory loss, which adds to the growing literature that obesity is primarily a neurodegenerative disease.

39. Halawi H, Khemani D, Eckert D, et al. Effects of liraglutide on weight, satiation, and gastric functions in obesity: a randomised, placebo-controlled trial. *Journal Lancet Gastroenterology & Hepatology* 2017; 2(12): 890-899.
DOI: 10.1016/S2468-1253(17)30285-6. PMID: 28958851

40. Uribarri J, Cai W, Woodward WC, et al. Elevated serum advanced glycation endproducts in obese indicate risk for the metabolic syndrome: a link between healthy and unhealthy obese. *Journal of Clinical Endocrinology & Metabolism* 2015; 100(5): 1957-1966.
DOI: 10.1210/jc.2014.3925. PMID: 25695886

41. Singh VP, Bali A, Singh N, Jaggi AS. Advanced Glycation end Products and diabetic Complications. *Korean Journal of Physiology & Pharmacology* 2014; 18(1): 1-14.
DOI: 10.4196/kjpp.2014.18.1.1. PMID: 24634591

42. Riviere S, Birlouez-Aragon I, Vellas B. Plasma protein glycation in Alzheimer's disease. *Glyconjugate Journal* 1998; 15(10): 1039-1042.
DOI: 10.1023/a:1006902428776. PMID: 10211709

43. Anwar A, Abruzzo PM, Pasha S, et al. Advanced glycation end products, dityrosine, and arginine transporter dysfunction in autism – a source of biomarkers for clinical diagnosis. *Molecular Autism* 2018; 9: 3. DOI: 10.1186/s13229-017-0183-3

# References

44. Colagiuri S. Glycated haemoglobin (HbA1c) for the diagnosis of diabetes mellitus - - practical implications. *Diabetes Research and Clinical Practice* 2011; 93(3): 312-313.
DOI: 10.1016/j.diabres.2011.06.025. PMID: 21820751

45. Alshwaiyat NM, Ahmad A, Hassan WMRW, Al-Jamal HANA-J. Association between obesity and iron deficiency (Review). *Experimental and Therapeutic Medicine* 2021; 22(5): 1268.
DOI: 10.3892/etm.2021.10703. PMID: 34594405

46. Soliman AT, De Sanctis V, Yassin M, Soliman N. Iron deficiency anemia and glucose metabolism. *Acta Biomedica* 2017; 88(1): 112-118. DOI: 10.23750/abm.v88i1.6049. PMID: 28467345

47. Hong CH, Falvey C, Harris TB, et al. Anemia and risk of dementia in older adults: findings from the Health ABC Study. *Neurology* 2013; 81(6): 528-533.
DOI: 10.1212/WNL.0b013e31829e701d. PMID: 23902706

48. Gunes S, Ekinci O, Celik T. Iron deficiency parameters in autism spectrum disorder: clinical correlates and associated factors. *Italian Journal of Pediatrics* 2017; 4: 86.
DOI: 10.1186/s13052-017-0407-3. PMID: 28934988

49. Lee A, Lingwood BE, Bjorkman ST, et al. Rapid loss of glutamine synthetase from astrocytes in response to hypoxia: implications for excitotoxicity. *Journal of Chemical Neuroanatomy* 2010; 39(3): 211-220 DOI: 10.1016/j.jchemneu.2009.12.002. PMID: 20034557

50. Norouzirad R, Gonzalez-Muniesa P, Ghasemi A. Hypoxia in Obesity and Diabetes: Potential Therapeutic Effects of Hyperoxia and Nitrite. *Oxidative Medicine and Cellular Longevity* 2017; 2017: 5350267. DOI: 10.1155/2017/5350267. PMID: 28607631

51. Catrina S-B, Zheng X. Hypoxia and hypoxia-inducible factors in diabetes and its complications. 2021; 64(4): 709-716.
DOI: 10.1007/s00125-021-05380-z. PMID: 33496820

52. Peers C, Pearson HA, Boyle JP. Hypoxia and Alzheimer's disease. *Essays in Biochemistry* 2007; 43: 153-164.
DOI: 10.1042/BSE0430153. PMID: 17705799

53. Burstyn I, Wang X, Yasui Y, et al. Autism spectrum disorders and fetal hypoxia in a population-based cohort: Accounting for missing exposures via Estimation-Maximization algorithm. *BMC Medical Research Methodology* 2011; 11:2. DOI: 10.1186/1471-2288-11-2. PMID: 21208442

54. Hammock EAD, Young LJ. Oxytocin, vasopressin, and pair bonding: implications for autism. *Philosophical Transactions R Soc Lond B Biol Sci* 2006; 361(1476): 2187-2198. DOI: 10.1098/rstb.2006.1939

Note: The authors found that oxytocin and vasopressin contributed to various social behaviours, including social recognition, communication, parental care, territorial aggression and social bonding.

55. Roussel R, Fezeu L, Bouby N, et al. Low Water Intake and Risk of New-Onset Hyperglycemia. *Diabetes Care* 2011; 34(12): 2551-2554. DOI: 10.2337/dc11.0652. PMID: 21994426

56. Bjorklund G, Kern JK, Urbina MA, et al. Cerebral hypoperfusion in autism spectrum disorder. *Acta Neurobiol Exp* 2018; 78(1): 21-29. PMID: 29694338

Note: This study found correlations between symptom scores and hypoperfusion in the brains of individuals diagnosed with autism, indicating that the greater the autism symptom pathology the greater the hypoperfusion (lack of water).

57. Wittbrodt MT, Millard-Stafford M. Dehydration Impairs Cognitive Performance: A Meta-analysis. *Medicine and Science in Sports and Exercise* 2018; 50(11): 2360-2368. DOI: 10.1249/MSS.0000000000001682. PMID: 29933347

Note: The authors found that the magnitude of dehydration was associated with the level of impairment in cognitive performance.

58. Tyagi MG, Parthiban KV. Vasopressin mediates neuroprotection in mice by stimulation of V1 vasopressin receptors: influence of P1-3 kinase and gap junction inhibitors. *Indian Journal of Experimental Biology* 2003; 41(6): 574-580. PMID: 152669002

# References

59. Ding C, Leow MK-S, Magkos F. Oxytocin in metabolic homeostasis: implications for obesity and diabetes. *Obesity Reviews* 2019; 20(1): 22-40. DOI: 10.1111/obr.12757. PMID: 30253045

60. Klement JJ, Ott V, Rapp K, et al. Oxytocin Improves B-Cell Responsivity and Glucose Tolerance in Healthy Men. *Diabetes* 2017; 66(2): 264-271. DOI: 10.2337/db16-0569. PMID: 27554476

61. Bernaerts S, Boets B, Bosmans G, Stayaert J, Alaerts K. Behavioral effects of multiple-dose oxytocin treatment in autism: a randomized, placebo-controlled trial with long-term follow-up. *Molecular Autism* 2020; 11: Article 6. DOI: 10.1186/s13229-020-0313-1. PMID: 31969977

62. Sayed N, Martens CA, Hsu WH. Arginine vasopressin increases glutamate release and intracellular Ca2+ concentration in hippocampal and cortical astrocytes through two distinct receptors. *Journal of Neurochemistry* 2007; 103(1): 229-237. DOI: 10.1111/j.1471-4519.04737.x. PMID: 17877638

63. Tan Y, Singhal SM, Harden SW, et al. Oxytocin Receptors Are Expressed by Glutamatergic Prefrontal Cortical Neurones That Selectively Modulate Social Recognition. *Journal of Neuroscience* 2019; 39(17): 3249-3263. DOI: 10.1523/JNEUROSCI.2944-18.2019. PMID: 30804095

64. Kim JS, Alderete TL, Chen Z, et al. Longitudinal associations of in utero and early life near-roadway air pollution with trajectories of childhood body mass index. *Environmental Health* 2018; 17(1): 64. DOI: 10.1186/s12940-018-0409-7. PMID: 30213262

65. Meroni G, Valerio A, Vezzoli M, et al. The relationship between air pollution and diabetes: A study on the municipalities of the Metropolitan City of Milan. *Diabetes Research and Clinical Practice* 2021; 174: 108748. DOI: 10.1016/j.diabres.2021.108748. PMID: 33713719

66. Moulton PV, Yang W. Air Pollution, Oxidative Stress and Alzheimer's Disease. *Journal of Environmental and Public Health* 2012; 2012: Article 1D 472751. DOI: 10.1155/2012/47251

67. Volk HE, Lurmann F, Penfold B, et al. Traffic-Related Air Pollution, Particulate Matter, and Autism. *JAMA Psychiatry* 2013; 70(1); 71-77. DOI: 10.1001/jamapsychiatry.2013.266

# Chapter 5: Sugar sickness syndrome one – Obesity

1. McClellan WS, Du Bois EF. Clinical Calorimetry: XLV. Prolonged Meat diets with a Study of Kidney Function and Ketosis. *Journal of Biological Chemistry* 1 July 1930.
DOI: 10.1016/S0021-9258(18)76842-7

Note: This rigorous year-long study shows that it is possible to live on a carbohydrate-free diet without ill effects. Ketogenic diets are increasingly used in specific medical conditions, such as epilepsy and some cancers. This was one of the most meticulously observed nutritional studies in history – every morsel of fat and meat that the subjects consumed was measured to the gram. Its historic importance has never been fully recognised.

2. Grasgruber P, Cacek J, Hrazdira E, Hrebickova S, Sebera M. Global Correlates of Cardiovascular risk: A Comparison of 158 Countries. *Nutrients* 2018; 10(4): 411.
DOI: 10.3390/nu10040411. PMID: 29587470

Note: The truth is finally out after half a century of obscurantism. These authors discovered that, regardless of the statistical method used, the trends identify high carbohydrate consumption as the dietary factor most consistently associated with the risk of cardiovascular disease.

3. Safiriyu AA, Semuyaba I, Lawal SK, et al. Comparative Study of the Effects of Metformin and Garlic Extract on hippocampal and Na+/K+ ATPase and Glutamine Synthetase Activities in Type 11 Diabetic Wistar Rat. *Journal of Biomedical Science and Engineering* 2018; 11: No 9. DOI: 10.4236/jbise.2018.119021

Note: This study demonstrated that metformin upgrades

glutamine synthetase, a finding that suggests its major influence may be in the brain. The health institutions have focused on the pancreas as the major energy-regulating gland in humans, but while it certainly plays a very important part, the science is now increasingly recognising that the key site of regulation is in the brain.

4. Yau PL, Javier DC, Ryan CM, Tsui WH, Ardekani BA, Convit A. Preliminary evidence for brain complications in obese adolescents with type 2 diabetes mellitus. *Diabetologia* 2010; 53(11): 2298-2306.
   DOI: 10.1007/s00125-010-1857-y. PMID: 20668831

   Note: This is an excellent study outlining serious lesions in the brains of obese/type 2 diabetic adolescents. The authors failed to connect this to overconsumption of sugars and suppressed glutamine synthetase, but it is a major contribution to the knowledge that obesity/type 2 diabetes pathology is neurodegenerative.

5. Maayan L, Hoogendoorn C, Sweat V, Convit A. Disinhibited eating in obese adolescents is associated with orbitofrontal volume reductions and executive dysfunction. *Obesity (Silver Spring)* 2011; 19(7): 1382-1387. DOI: 10.1038/oby.2011.15. PMID: 21350433

   Note: This alarming 2011 study on reduced brain volume in obese young people should have raised a storm across the globe but no such reaction occurred. Parents were becoming increasingly immune to obesity in their children, and those who should have raised the neuropathology alarm did not do so.

6. Courcoulas AP, Yanovski SZ, Bonds D, et al. Long-term Outcomes of Bariatric Surgery: A National Institutes of Health Symposium. *JAMA Surgery* 2014; 149(12): 1323-1329 .
   DOI: 10.1001/jamasurg 2014.2440. PMID: 25271405

7. Pories WJ, Swanson MS, MacDonald KG, et al. Who would have thought it? An operation proves to be the most effective therapy for adult-onset diabetes mellitus. *Annals of Surgery* 1995; 222(3): 339-352.

DOI: 10.1097/000000658-199509000-00011. PMID: 7677463

Note: This is a truly astonishing study that shows lowering blood glucose in obesity, via gut reduction, reverses type 2 diabetes, and that the improved glucose control begins long before the weight loss occurs. Therefore increased blood glucose concentration (hyperglycaemia) emerges as the most significant index in both obesity and type 2 diabetes.

8. Handley JD, Willians DM, Caplin S, et al. Changes in Cognitive Function Following Bariatric Surgery: a Systematic Review. *Journal Obesity Surgery* 2016; 26(10): 2530-2537. DOI: 10.1007/s11695-016-2312-z. PMID: 27468905

Note: The context of this research was the known direct association between increased body mass and reduced cognitive function. The authors found in a systematic review of 18 research papers that 'significant and rapid weight loss' as a result of bariatric surgery was 'associated with prompt and sustained improvements in cognitive function'. This included 'memory, executive function and cognitive control'.

9. Wong M. Mammalian Target of Rapamycin (mTOR) Pathway in Neurological Diseases. *Biomedical Journal* 1013; 36(2): 40-50. DOI: 10.4103/2319-4170.110365. PMID: 23644232

Note: This important study connects excess energy (characteristic of late-modern excess-sugar-consuming humans) to neurological and cognitive malfunction.

10. Mao Z, Zhang W. Role of mTOR in Glucose and Lipid Metabolism. *International Journal of Molecular Sciences* 2018; 19(7): 2043. DOI: 10.3390/ijms19072043. PMID: 30011848

Note: mTOR is a major high-energy pathway that is dysregulated in obesity and diabetes. This dysregulation is opposed by rapamycin.

11. Garcia-Ptacek S, Faxen-Irving G, Cermakova P, et al. Body mass index in dementia. *European Journal of Clinical Nutrition* 2014; 68(11): 1204-1209 DOI: 10.1038/ejcn.2014.199. PMID: 25271014

Note: The authors showed that in younger adults, higher BMIs are associated with impaired cognition. Overweight and obesity in middle age were linked to increased future dementia risk in old age. However, when examined in old age, higher BMIs were associated with better cognition and decreased mortality. This is one of the most interesting paradoxes in human energy regulation. In old age a higher BMI with increased lean tissue protects against dementia by muscle consumption of glucose and reduced levels of circulating glucose, thereby facilitating glutamine synthetase and improving glucose energy transport into the brain.

12. Pagani M, Barsotti N, Bertero A, et al. mTOR-related synaptic pathology causes autism spectrum disorder-associated functional hyperconnectivity. *Nature Communications* 2021; 12(1): 6084. DOI: 10.1038/s41467-021-26131-z. PMID: 34667149

13. Kahathuduwa CN, West BD, Blume J, et al. The risk of overweight and obesity in children with autism spectrum disorders: A systematic review and meta-analysis. *Obesity Review* 2019; 20(12): 1667-1679. DOI: 10.1111/obr.12933. PMID: 31595678

14. Kahn BB, Flier JS. Obesity and insulin resistance. *Journal of Clinical Investigations* 2000; 1064(4): 473-481. DOI: 10.1172/JCI10842

Note: The authors found that insulin resistance and hyperinsulinaemia, in addition to being caused by obesity, can contribute to the development of obesity. Insulin resistance and hyperinsulinaemia are normally associated with type 2 diabetes. This study beautifully confirms that these two ailments are essentially similar excess-sugar-driven conditions. Yes, fats can influence insulin resistance and consequent hyperinsulinaemia, but this is driven by high levels of circulating glucose as the initiating event.

15. Stern M. Insulin signaling and autism. *Frontiers in Endocrinology* 2011; 2: 54. DOI: 10.3389/fendo.2011.00054. PMID: 22649376

# Chapter 6: Sugar sickness syndrome two – Type 2 diabetes

1. World Health Organization. Diabetes: Key facts. 16 September 2022. www.who.int/news-room/fact-sheets/detail/diabetes (accessed 9 March 2023)

2. Wild S, Roglic G, Green A, et al. Global prevalence of diabetes: estimates for the year 2000 and projections for 2030. *Diabetes Care* 2004; 27(5): 1047-53. DOI: 10.2337/diacare.27.5.1047

3. Zimmet PZ. Diabetes and its drivers: the largest epidemic in human history? *Clin Diabetes Endocrinol* 2017; 3: 1. DOI: 10.1186/s40842-016-0039-3

   Note: The author compares the epidemic of 'diabesity' to the Black Death of 1346-1353.

4. Rennie J, Fraser T. The Islets of Langerhans in Relation to Diabetes. *Biochemistry Journal* 1907; 2(1-2): 7-19. DOI: 10.1042/bj0020007. PMID: 16742063

   Note: An excellent early study of the pancreas as a modulator of glucose control.

5. Brostoff JM, Keen H, Brostoff JA. A diabetic life before and after the insulin era. *Diabetologia* 2007; 50: 1351-1353. DOI 10.1007/s00125-007-0641-0

6. Young FG. Claude Bernard and the Discovery of Glycogen. *British Medical Journal* 1957; 1(5033): 1431-1437. DOI: 10.1136/bmj.1.5033.1431. PMID: 13436813

7. Paton DN. The Effect of Adrenaline on Sugar and Nitrogen Excretion in the Urine of Birds. *Journal of Physiology* 1904; 3032(1): 59-64. DOI: 10.1113/jphysiol.1904.sp001065.

   Note: As early as 1904 D Noel Paton shows that if the body (and therefore the brain) is deprived of energy in diabetes, proteins are degraded and ammonia released.

8. Hirata Y, Nomura K, Senga Y, et al. Hyperglycemia induces skeletal

muscle atrophy via a WWP1/KLF15 axis. *Journal of Clinical Investigation Insight* 2019; 4(4): e124952.
DOI: 10.1172/jci.insight.124952. PMID: 30830866

Note: The authors discovered that diabetes mellitus was associated with various disorders of the locomotor system including the decline in mass of skeletal muscle. This is a wonderful study linking muscle degradation to excess circulating glucose. How does that link work? Excess systemic glucose inhibits the brain's glucose pump, glutamine synthetase. The energy-hungry brain organises degradation of muscle which is transported to the liver and converted to glucose (gluconeogenesis). The new glucose adds to the problem, further increasing muscle degradation and the cycle repeats.

9. Lopez Teros MT, Ramirez FA, Aleman-Mateo H. Hyperinsulinemia is associated with loss of appendicular skeletal muscle mass at 4.6-year follow-up in older men and women. *Journal of Clinical Nutrition* 2015; 34(5): 931-936.
DOI: 10.1016/j.clnu.2014.09.022. PMID: 2543394

Note: This excellent study confirms that hyperinsulinaemia degrades muscle – this is a signal of hyperinsulinaemia suppression of glutamine synthetase in glia, brain energy deficiency and consequent creation of glucose in the liver, an attempt to increase blood glucose levels, adding to the problem, although the authors did not make that critical connection.

10. Goodheart S. Meet the Creature that Eats its Own Brain. Goodheart's Extreme Science. Posted 27 January 2010.
https://goodheartextremescience.wordpress.com/2010/01/27/meet-the-creature-that-eats-its-own-brain/

Note: This is an excellent article on the sea squirt brain.

11. Ola MS, Hosoya K-I, LaNoue KF. Influence of insulin on glutamine synthetase in the muller cells of the retina. *Metabolic Brain Disease* 2011; 26(3): 195-202.
DOI: 10.1007/s11011-011-9245-y. PMID: 21626103

Note: One of the most significant studies outlining how excess insulin (hyperinsulinaemia) in modern excess-sugar-consuming humans impairs the brain's glucose pump, yet cited by only two subsequent studies in a decade – shameful!

12. Li C, Buettger C, Kwagh J, et al. A signaling role of glutamine in insulin secretion. *Journal of Metabolism and Bioenergetics* 2004: 279(14): 13393-13401. DOI: 10.1074/jbc.M311502200. PMID: 14736887

Note: This wonderful study from Pennsylvania University, USA, shows that glutamine (and therefore glutamine synthetase which converts glutamate to glutamine) plays a role in insulin control of glucose metabolism. This beautifully confirms the mutual and interdependent metabolism of glutamine synthetase and insulin – energy income regulates the governor (insulin), the governor regulates the fuel pump (glutamine synthetase) and the fuel pump regulates the governor, a triad which oversees all energy income and expenditure.

13. Reid J, MacDougall AI, Andrews MM. Aspirin and Diabetes Mellitus. *British Medical Journal* 1957; 2(5053): 1071-1074. DOI: 10.1136/bmj.2.5053.1071. PMID: 1342052

Note: This is an historic study from Glasgow Western Infirmary – a trio of researchers first identified diabetes as an inflammatory disease.

14. Shoelson SE, Lee J, Goldfine AB. Inflammation and insulin resistance. *Journal of Clinical Investigation* 2006; 116(7): 1793-1801. DOI: 10.1172/JCI29069. PMID: 16823477

15. de Cristobal J, Moro MA, Davalos A, et al. Neuroprotective effect of aspirin by inhibition of glutamate release after permanent focal cerebral ischaemia in rats. *Journal of Neurochemistry* 2001; 79(2): 456-459. DOI: 10.1046/j.1471-4519.2001.00600x. PMID: 11677274

16. UK Prospective Diabetes Study (UKPDS) Group. Effect of intensive blood-glucose control with metformin in overweight patients with type 2 diabetes (UKPDS 34). *Lancet* 1998; 352(9131): 854-865. PMID: 9742977

17. Safiriyu A, Semuyaba I, Lawal S, Buhari MO, et al. Comparative Study of the Effects of Metformin and Garlic Extract on the Hippocampal Na+/K+ ATPase, Ca+ATPase and Glutamate Synthetase Activities in Type 11 Diabetic Wistar Rats. *Journal of Biomedical Science and Engineering* 2018; 11(9): 254-262. DOI: 10.4236/jbise.2018.119021

Note: This is an historic study giving us new understanding of the actions of metformin and indicating that type 2 diabetes is a centrally modulated disease that impairs cognition via suppression of glutamine synthetase yet it has been cited only once since publication in 2018.

18. Pories WJ, Swanson MS, MacDonald KG, et al. Who would have thought it? An operation proves to be the most effective therapy for adult-onset diabetes mellitus. *Annals of Surgery* 1995; 222(3): 339-352. DOI: 10.1097/000000658-199509000-00011. PMID: 7677463

# Chapter 7: Sugar sickness syndrome three – Alzheimer's disease

1. Fisher Center for Alzheimer's Research Foundation, Rockefeller University, USA. www.rockefeller.edu/research/interdisciplinary-centers/cenzach/ (accessed 9 March 2022)

2. Alzheimer's Disease International. Dementia Statistics. *World Alzheimer Report 2015.* www.alzint.org/about/dementia-facts-figures/dementia-statistics/ (accessed 9 March 2023)

3. Multiple Dementia Collaborators Forecasting. Estimation of the global prevalence of dementia in 2019 and forecasted prevalence in 2050: an analysis of the Global Burden of Disease Study 2019. *Lancet* 2022; 7(2): E105-E125. DOI: 10.1016/S2468-2667(21)00249-8.

4. Mayo Clinic. Alzheimer's stages: How the disease progresses. *Mayo Clinic News* April 2021. www.mayoclinic.org/diseases-conditions/alzheimers-disease/in-depth/alzheimers-stages/art-20048448 (accessed 13 March 2023)

5. Nguyen TT, Ta QTH, Nguyen TKO, et al. Type 3 Diabetes and Its Role Implications in Alzheimer's Disease. *International Journal of Molecular Science* 2020; 21(9): 3165. DOI: 10.3390/ijms21093165. PMID: 32365816

6. Mosconi L, Mitsur R, Switalski R, et al. FDG-PAT changes in brain glucose metabolism from normal cognition to pathologically verified Alzheimer's disease. *European Journal of Nuclear Medicine and Molecular Imaging* 2009; 36(5): 811-822. DOI: 10.1007/s00259-008-1039-z. PMID: 19142633

Note: This alarming study demonstrated that declining brain metabolic rate occurs many years before clinical symptoms of dementia appear and pathological diagnosis of Alzheimer's disease.

7. Robinson SR. Neuronal expression of glutamine synthetase in Alzheimer's disease indicates a profound impairment of metabolic interactions with astrocytes. *Neurochemistry International* 2000 Apr;36(4-5):471-82. DOI: 10.1016/s0197-0186(99)00150-3. PMID: 10733015

Note: This important study indicated that in Alzheimer's disease reduced glutamine synthetase cycling in glia stimulated its appearance in neurones – this strongly suggests that when the G/G cycle is deficient in glia (astrocytes), neurones deprived of energy attempt to activate the cycle in a futile recovery response.

8. Serrano-Pozo A, Mielke ML, Gomez-Isla T, et al. Reactive Glia not only associates with Plaques but also Parallels Tangles in Alzheimer's Disease. *American Journal of Pathology* 2011; 179(3): 1373-1384. DOI: 10.1016/j.ajpath.2011.05.047. PMID: 21777559

Note: This is an important study linking amyloid deposition to reactive glia. Gliosis is a fibrous proliferation of glia in injured areas of the brain – an attempt to increase glutamine synthetase action, when compromised.

9. Harris S. Hyperinsulinism and Dysinsulinism. *Journal of the American Medical Association* 1924; 83(10): 729-733. DOI: 10.1001/jama.1924.02660100003002.

# References

Note: Ground-breaking study from a century ago, linking hyperinsulinaemia to hunger, a perspective now confirmed in the knowledge that excess consumption of refined sugar suppresses the enzyme glutamine synthetase, deprives the brain of energy, appetite hormones are released and the cycle repeats. A century later this understanding is still not recognised by the health institutions, governments and of course the food/sugar lobby.

10. Luchsinger JA. Hyperinsulinemia and risk of Alzheimer disease. *Neurology* 2004; 63(7): 1187-1192.
DOI: 10.1212/01.wnl.0000140292.04932.87. PMID: 154775336

Note: The author found that hyperinsulinaemia was associated with a higher risk of Alzheimer's disease and decline in memory – confirmation of Seale Harris' work, a century on.

11. Stern M. Insulin signaling and autism. *Frontiers in Endocrinology* 2011; 2: 54. DOI: 10.3389/fendo.2011.00054. PMID: 22649376

Note: This is a seminal study in autism indicating impaired insulin signalling as a key factor and indicating a likely influence of sugar metabolism, shared with Alzheimer's disease. This study has been almost entirely overlooked by the autism scientific community. Two cognitively impaired conditions share a common pathway, one at the beginning of and one in later life.

12. Kurochkin IV, Goto S. Alzheimer's beta-amyloid peptide specifically interacts with and is degraded by insulin degrading enzyme. *FEBS Letters* 1994; 345(1): 33-37.
DOI: 10.1016/0014-5793(94)00387-4. PMID: 8194595

Note: An important early study showing that excess insulin (hyperinsulinaemia) prevents amyloid degrading activity – via corralling IDE and contributing to Alzheimer's disease.

13. Askok A, Singh N, Chaudhary S, et al. Retinal degeneration and Alzheimer's disease: An evolving link. *Int J Mol Sci* 2020; 21(19): 7290. DOI: 10.3390/ijms21197290

14. Cheung CY, Mok V, Foster PJ, et al. Retinal imaging in Alzheimer's disease. *Journal of Neurology, Neurosurgery and Psychiatry* 2021;

92(9): 983-994. DOI: 10.1136/jnnp-2020-325347. PMID: 34108266

Note: This is an excellent study demonstrating that, via retinal imaging, the eye is the first organ to signal cognitive impairments in Alzheimer's disease.

15. Amieva H, Ouvrard C, Meillon, et al. Death, Depression, Disability, and Dementia associated with Self-reported Hearing Problems: A 25-Year Study. *Journals of Gerontology: Series A* 2018; 73(10): 1383-1389. DOI: 10.1093/gerona/glx250. PMID: 29304204

Note: This important study links hearing loss to dementia. Not referenced by the authors is the knowledge that impaired glutamine synthetase, universal in modern sugar consuming humans, is critical to information/energy coupling in the auditory metabolic pathway.

16. Nordang L, Cestreicher E, Arnold W, Anniko M. Glutamate is the afferent neurotransmitter in the human cochlea. *Acta Oto-Laryngologica* 2000; 120(3): 359-362.
DOI: 10.1080/000164800750000568. PMID: 10894409

Note: The authors described glutamate as the most important afferent neurotransmitter in the auditory system and confirmed the role of glutamatergic transmission in the auditory pathway, and the key role of glutamine synthetase in hearing.

17. Roberts RO, Christianson TJH, Kremers WK, et al. Association between olfactory dysfunction and amnestic mild cognitive impairment and Alzheimer disease dementia. *Journal of the American Medical Association Neurology* 2016; 73(1): 93-101. DOI: 10.1001/jamaneurol.2015.2952. PMID: 26569387

Note: The authors found significant connections between impaired olfaction (smell) and the progression to Alzheimer's disease.

18. Steinbach S, Hundt A, Vaitl A, et al. Taste in mild cognitive impairment and Alzheimer's disease. *Journal of Neurology* 2010; 257(2): 238-246. DOI: 10.1007/s00415-009-5300-6. PMID: 19727902

Note: The authors concluded that there was a significant

reduction in total taste scores on either side of the tongue between controls and mild cognitively impaired and Alzheimer's patients.

19. Tsujimoto T, Imai K, Kanda S, et al. Sweet taste disorder and vascular complications in patients with abnormal glucose tolerance. *International Journal of Cardiology* 2016; 221: 637-641. DOI: 10.1016/j.ijcard.2016.07.062. PMID: 27423082

Note: Of particular interest was that the sweet taste disorder was closely connected to vascular complications which are associated with diabetic retinopathy – a critical measure of glutamine synthetase impairment.

20. Vandenbeuch A, Kinnamon SAC. Glutamate: Tastant and Neuromodulator in Taste Buds. *Advances in Nutrition* 1016; 7(4): 8235-8275. DOI: 10.3945/an.115.01.011304

Note: Taste, like all sensory perception pathways, requires optimal glutamatergic transmission, so that information and energy can be couple.

21. Benedetti F, Vighetti S, Ricco C, et al. Pain threshold and tolerance in Alzheimer's disease. *Pain* 1999; 80(1-2): 377-382. DOI: 10.1016/s0304-3959(98)00228-0. PMID: 10204751

Note: Increased pain threshold is a key cognitive pathway linking information impairment with reduced sensory perception.

22. Wozniak KM, Roja C, Wu Y, Slusher BS. The role of glutamate signaling in pain processes and its regulation by GCP 11 inhibition. *Current Medicinal Chemistry* 2012; 19(9): 1323-1334. DOI: 10.2174/092986712799462630. PMID: 22304711

Note: This excellent study indicates the role of glutamate (and therefore of glutamine synthetase) in pain transmission.

23. Wei J, Karsenty G. An overview of the metabolic functions of osteocalcin. *Reviews in Endocrine and Metabolic Disorders* 2015; 16(2): 93-98. DOI: 10.1007/s11154-014-9307-7

Note: This is an important review of the bone hormone osteocalcin in energy (glucose) regulation. This connects to the recognised link of dysderegulated energy metabolism in type 2 diabetes and increased risk of bone fractures.

24. Fernandes TAP, Goncalves LML, Brito JAA. Relationships between Bone Turnover and Energy Metabolism. *Journal of Diabetes Research* 2017; 2017: 9021314. DOI: 10.1155/2017/9021314. PMID: 28695134

25. Lekkala A, Taylor EA, Hunt HB, Donnelly E. Effects of Diabetes on Bone Material Properties. *Current Osteoporosis Reports* 2019; 17(6): 455-464. DOI: 10.1007/s11914-00538-6

26. Zhou T, Yang Y, Chen Q, Xie L. Glutamine Metabolism is Essential for Stemness of Bone Marrow Mesenchymal Stem Stells and bone Homeostasis. *Stem Cells International* 2019; 2019: Article 8928934. DOI: 10.1155/2019/8928934. PMID: 31611919

Note: This is a Chinese study linking impaired glutamine metabolism (and therefore reduced glutamine synthetase integrity) to bone diseases.

27. Ekhlaspour L, Baskaran C, Campoverde KJ, et al. Bone Density in Adolescents and Young Adults with Autism Spectrum Disorders. *Journal of Autism and Developmental Disorders* 2016; 46(11): 3387-3391. DOI: 10.1007/s10803-016-2871-9. PMID: 27491424

Note: This deeply concerning Harvard University study links the risk of bone fracture to cognitive impairments. Considering this paper's importance it is disappointing to see it has been cited just 12 times since 2016.

# Chapter 8: Sugar sickness syndrome zero – Autism spectrum disorders

1. University of Cambridge. Autism prevalence in China. University of Cambridge News: Research Collaboration of University of Cambridge with China Disabled Persons' Federation, and Chinese

# References

University of Hong Kong. 18th April 2013. www.cam.ac.uk/news/autism-prevalence-in-china-0 (accessed 13 March 2023)

2. Hamed NO, Al-Ayadhi L, Osman MA, et al. Understanding the roles of glutamine synthetase, glutaminase, and glutamate decarboxylase autoantibodies in imbalanced excitatory/inhibitory neurotransmission as etiological mechanisms of autism. *Journal of Psychiatry and Clinical Neurosciences* 2018; 72(5): 361-373. DOI: 10.1111/pcn.12639. PMID: 29356297

Note: Impaired glutamate/glutamine cycling is a marker of all excess-sugar-driven metabolic (energy dysregulation) diseases. This study under the auspices of the Ethical Committee of the Faculty of Medicine, King Saud University, Riyadh, Saudi Arabia, is of immense importance. Increased excitotoxicity is indicative of increased glutamate and impaired glutamine synthetase. Glutamate is highly toxic and must be converted to glutamine to avoid neurotoxic damage and death of neurones. Presumably because this study was conducted in the Middle East, it has received only two citations globally.

3. Sokol DK, Chen D, Farlow MR, et al. High levels of Alzheimer beta-amyloid precursor protein (APP) in children with severely autistic behavior and aggression. *Journal of Child Neurology* 2006; 21(6): 444-449.
DOI: 10.1177/08830738060210062201. PMID: 16948926

Note: This alarming study links beta-amyloid accumulation in autistic children, usually associated with Alzheimer's disease. Aggression is also recognised in Alzheimer's disease.

4. Vogelstein F. Epilepsy's Big Fat Miracle. *New York Times* 17 November 2010. www.nytimes.com/2010/11/21/magazine/21Epilepsy-t.html

Note: This is a fascinating article on epilepsy and controlling it via a carbohydrate-free diet. From well over 100 seizures a day, Fred's son Sam experienced fewer than six. What Sam's father Fred could not have known is that the driving force of epileptic fits is excess glutamate, and reducing carbohydrate and sugars reduces oxidative degradation of glutamine synthetase, thereby improving glutamate/glutamine cycling and lowering toxic levels of glutamate in the brain.

5. Wright J. The link between epilepsy and autism, explained. *Spectrum* 21 October 2019. www.spectrumnews.org/news/the-link-between-epilepsy-and-autism-explained/

Note: Jessica Wright noted that about 10% of persons with autism have epilepsy and that the number from other studies ranges from 2 to 46%.

6. Meldrum BS. The role of glutamate in epilepsy and other CNS disorders. *Neurology* 1994; 44(11 Suppl 8): S14-S23. PMID: 7970002

Note: This study outlines glutamate (and therefore impaired glutamine synthetase) as a major influence on epilepsy. This is an advance in the understanding of how excess circulating sugars (hyperglycaemia) along with hyperinsulinaemia suppress this vital enzyme.

7. Jaber MA. Dental caries experience, oral health and treatment needs of patients with autism. *Journal of Applied Oral Science* 2011; 19(3): 212-217.
DOI: 10.1590/S1678-77572011000300006. PMID: 21625735

8. Price WA. *Nutrition and Physical Degeneration 8th Edition.* Price-Pottenger Nutrition Foundation; 2009.

9. Bagramian RA, Garcia-Godoy F, Volpe AR. The global increase in dental caries. A pending public health crisis. *American Journal of Dentistry* 2009; 22(1): 3-8. PMID: 19281105

10. Wissing C, Rougier H, Crevecoeur I, et al. Isotopic evidence for dietary ecology of late Neanderthals in North-Western Europe. *Quaternary International* 2016; 411(A): 327-349.
DOI: 10.1016/j.quaint.2015.09.091

11. Molinaro A, Micheletti S, Rossi A, et al. Autistic-Like Features in Visually Impaired Children: A Review of Literature and Directions for Future Research. *Brain Sciences* 2020; 10(8): 507.
DOI: 10.3390/brainsci10080507. PMID: 32752249

# References

Note: This revealing study indicates a form of 'sugar blindness' in the autistic science community. In modern human populations sugar consumption vastly exceeds that of previous generations. Sugar-induced blindness (retinopathy) accounts for around 80% of blind persons globally. Vision is one of the key information pathways involved in the human mind and is critical in the theory of mind. Refined sugars are teratogenic (damaging to the foetus). The failure to connect foetal and postnatal visual impairments to refined sugar consumption is an indictment of the bioscientific community.

12. Torres-Espinola FJ, Berglund SK, Garcia S, et al. Visual evoked potentials in offspring born to mothers with overweight, obesity and gestational diabetes. *Plos One* 2018: e203754. DOI: 10.1371/journal.pone.0203754. PMID: 30208080

Note: The relationship between overweight and neurodevelopmental injury is included – vital information for prospective parents, but largely hidden from the public.

13. Jure R. Seeing connections between autism and blindness. *Spectrum* 12 November 2019. www.spectrumnews.org/opinion/viewpoint/seeing-connections-between-autism-and-blindness/

Note: In this excellent article, Jure explored the remarkable connection between autism and visual impairments. He noted that, to the seasoned eye, the similarities between blindism and autism were striking.

14. Hammock EAD, Young LJ. Oxytocin, vasopressin, and pair bonding: implications for autism. *Philosophical Transactions R Soc London B Biol Sci* 2006; 361(1476): 2187-2198. DOI: 10.1098/rstb.2006.1939

Note: The authors stated that oxytocin and vasopressin contributed to various social behaviours, including social recognition, communication, parental care, territorial aggression and social bonding.

15. Roussel R, Fezeu L, Bouby N, et al. Low Water Intake and Risk of New-Onset Hyperglycemia. *Diabetes Care* 2011; 34(12): 2551-2554.

DOI: 10.2337/dc11.0652. PMID: 21994426

16. Bjorklund G, Kern JK, Urbina MS, et al. Cerebral hypoperfusion in autism spectrum disorder. *Acta Neurobiol Exp (Wars)* 2018; 78(1): 21-29. PMID: 29694338

   Note: This study found correlations between symptom scores for autism and hypoperfusion in the brains of individuals diagnosed with autism spectrum disorders, indicating that the greater the autism symptom pathology the greater the problem with brain hydration. We should note that the most universal and toxic factor for dehydration, in body and brain, is that of excess circulating glucose.

17. Bernaerts S, Boets B, Bosmans G, et al. Behavioral effects of multiple-dose oxytocin treatment in autism: a randomized, placebo-controlled trial with long-term follow-up. *Molecular Autism* 2020; 11(1): 6.
   DOI: 10.1186/s13229-020-0313-1. PMID: 31969977

18. Sayed N, Martens CA, Hsu WH. Arginine vasopressin increases glutamate release and intracellular Ca2+ concentration in hippocampal and cortical astrocytes through two distinct receptors. *Journal of Neurochemistry* 2007; 103(1): 229-237.
   DOI: 10.1111/j.1471-4519.04737x. PMID: 17877638

19. Tan Y, Singhal SM, Harden SW, et al. Oxytocin Receptors Are Expressed by Glutamatergic Prefrontal Cortical Neurones That Selectively Modulate Social Recognition. *Journal of Neuroscience* 2019; 39(17): 3249-3263.
   DOI: 10.1523/JNEUROSCI.2944-18.2019. PMID: 30804095

20. Crider A, Pillai A. Estrogen Signaling as a Therapeutic Target in Neurodevelopmental Disorders. *Journal of Pharmacology and Experimental Therapeutics* 2017; 360(1): 48-58.
   DOI: 10.1124/jpet.116.237412. PMID: 27789681.

   Note: Oestrogens are protective in neurodevelopmental disorders including autism. We also know that oestrogens protect against excess sugar oxidative neurodegeneration in the brain.

21. Blustein T, Devidze N, Choleris E, et al. Oestradiol up-regulates glutamine synthetase mRNA and protein expression in the hypothalamus and hippocampus: implications for a role of hormonally responsive glia in amino acid neurotransmission. *Journal of Neuroendocrinology* 2006; 18(9): 692-702. DOI: 10.1111/j.1365-2826.01466x. PMID: 16879168

Note: Upgrading glutamine synthetase is a major counter to all the metabolic (energy dysregulation) diseases – the sugar sickness syndromes that are currently degrading human physiology and cognition. The glial cells are ground zero in this developing tragedy.

22. Schulster M, Bernie AM, Ramasamy R. The role of estradiol in male reproductive function. *Asian Journal of Andrology* 2016; 18(3): 435-440. DOI: 10.4103/1008.682X.173932. PMID: 26908066

23. Baron-Cohen S, Tsompanidis A, Auyeung B, et al. Foetal oestrogens and autism. *Molecular Psychiatry* 2020; 25(11): 2970-2978. DOI: 10.1038/s41380-019-0454-9. PMID: 31358906

Note: The authors found increased production of oestrogens in autism – in both males and females. It seems to be more fruitful in girls than boys which may indicate a degree of male resistance to extra oestrogens.

## Chapter 9: Honey and its bioflavonoids

1. Bakkar RT. Dinosaur feeding behaviour and the origins of flowering plants. *Nature* 1978; 274: 661-663.

2. Smerilli A, Balzano S, Maselli M, et al. Antioxidant and Photoprotection Networking in the Coastal Diatom *Skeletonema marinoi*. *Antioxidants* 2019; 8(6): 154. DOI: 10.3390/antiox8060154. PMID: 31159429

Note: This important Danish/Italian study established that the source of the honey bioflavonoids that protect the human brain from sugar-induced neurodegeneration, and are found in ancient microalgae, is that of light energy. In other words, the very origins of plant and animate life, via elaboration of sugar fuels (photosynthesis), is also the driver of the creation of the biomolecules that protect animate life from light-driven oxidative degradation. There could be no sweeter paradox in the evolution of species.

3. Robertson DI, Smith GJ, Alberte RS. Glutamine synthetase in marine algae: new surprises from an old enzyme. *Journal of Psychology* 2001; 37(5): 793-795. DOI: 10.1046/j.1529-8817.2001.01057.x

Note: This study showed that ancient algae (from up to 1.7 billion years ago) expressed glutamine synthetase (and which was later conserved as the enzyme of cognition in all animate species including humans, around 400 million years ago at the birth of primitive nervous systems). The conclusions are that glutamine synthetase catalyses the formation of glutamine from ammonia and glutamate and that recent biochemical and molecular data suggest that this type of enzyme is broadly distributed among the algae.

4. Grainger D. A votre sante? *Lancet* 2000; 356(9224): 92. DOI: 10.1016/S0140-6736(00)02467-3

5. Blatt J, Roces F. Haemolymph sugar levels in foraging honeybees (Apis mellifera carnica): dependence on metabolic rate and in vivo rates of trehalose synthesis. *Journal of Experimental Biology* 2001; 204(Pt 15): 2709-2716.
DOI: 10.1242/jeb.204.15.2709. PMID: 11533121

Note: This is an astonishing study that showed the honeybee brain during foraging functions efficiently although carrying a sugar load in its circulation that should overwhelm glutamine synthetase and cause an inflammatory cascade that destroys its neurones, but does not.

6. Seal R. Breakfast of champions: Albert Einstein's fried eggs in honey. *Guardian* 25 April 2015. www.theguardian.com/lifeandstyle/2015/apr/25/breakfast-of-champions-albert-einstein-fried-eggs-in-honey (accessed 9 April 2023)

7. Dyer AG, Greentree AD, Garcia JE, et al. Einstein, von Frisch and the

honeybee: a historical letter comes to light. *Journal of Comparative Physiology: Neuroethology, Sensory, Neural and Behavioral Physiology* 2021; 207(4): 449-456. DOI: 10.1007/s00359-021-6. PMID: 33970340

8. BBC goodfood. Is honey good for you? BBC Good Food Website. Article reviewed on 24 June 2019. www.bbcgoodfood.com/ howto/guide/is-honey-good-for-you (accessed 12 March 2023)

9. Crittenden AN. The Importance of Honey Consumption in Human Evolution. *Food and Foodways* 2011; 19(4): 257-273. DOI: 10.1080/07409710.2011.630618

Note: This is one of the most seminal studies on human cognition in evolution. No other food/fuel existed or exists that could generate the leap in cognition, communication and language compared to honey in terms of controlled energy density, genetic fecundity and accessibility. What Alyssa Crittenden has contributed is a breakthrough in our understanding of how early prehumans (hominins) became *Homo sapiens* in the previous 200,000 years and what could have been the catalyst in that exponential intellectual leap forward. Only honey fulfils that role.

10. Goren-Inbar N. Evidence of Hominin Control of Fire at Gesher Benot Ya'aqov, Israel. *Science* 2004; 304(5671): 725-727. DOI: 10.1126/science.1095443

Note: This study shows the wide variety of food resources and use of fire from 750,000 years ago.

11. Wrangham R. Control of fire in the Palaeolithic: Evaluating the Cooking Hypothesis. *Current Anthropology* 2017; 58: s16. DOI: org/10.1086/692113

Note: Richard Wrangham claims that, unlike other animals, *Homo sapiens* has evolved an obligation to include cooked food in the diet. This paper is an interesting study of the notion that increased energy gain from cooking is a key factor in the increased brain size in the period starting 2.5 million years ago. There is little doubt that this energy gain, along with reduced gut size, would have been a significant benefit in the advance of hominid species. With respect to the brain this is problematic.

Protein is not a fuel in the brain. Control of fire would have benefited our developing species because fire was used to calm honeybees during collection of honey, and honey is emerging as the critical energy-dense (but controlled) brain fuel that may have been the catalyst in the cognitive leap of our species around 200,000 years ago.

12. Alpers DH. Is glutamine a unique fuel for small intestinal cells? *Current Opinion in Gastroenterology* 2000; 16(2): 155. DOI: 10.1097/00001574-200003000-00010. PMID: 17024034

Note: Alpers concludes that 'The major fuels for the small intestinal mucosa are amino acids (glutamine, glutamate, aspartate), whereas glucose and fatty acids are of much less importance'.

13. Perry GH, Dominy NJ, Claw KC, et al. Diet and the evolution of human amylase gene copy number variation. *Nature Genetics* 2007; 39: 1256-1260. DOI: 10.1038/ng2123

Note: This excellent study shows that the leap forward of brain growth in our ancestors is related to starch consumption and increased amylase function which enhanced glucose uptake. This of course contrasts with modern refined sugar consumption that overloads the brain's fuel pump (glutamine synthetase) and deprives the brain of glucose energy – key to the major metabolic (energy dysregulation) diseases.

14. Wheeler MM, Robinson GE. Diet-dependent gene expression in honey bees vs. sucrose or high fructose corn syrup. *Nature Scientific Reports* 2014; 4: Article 5726. DOI: 10.1038/srep05726. PMID: 25034029

Note: This study was a breakthrough in understanding the differences between the metabolism of honey and refined sugars as expressed by their genetic fertility. It quite beautifully nails the nonsense articulated by the major health institutions and professionals that honey is no different to refined sugars in the same quantity. Honey activates hundreds of genes that refined sugars do not.

15. Shpigler HY, Saul MC, Corona F, Black L, Ahmed AC, Shao SD, Robinson GE. Deep evolutionary conservation of autism-related genes. *Proceedings of the National Academy of Sciences* 2017; 114(36): 9653-9658. DOI: 10.1073/pnas.1708127114. PMID: 28760967

Note: This is a brilliant and revealing study of the genetic biology of social behaviour shared by honeybees and humans. It also relates to the study above (reference 14) and the role of honeybee genetics in response to honey and refined sugars. The authors showed that their results demonstrated deep conservation for genes implicated in autism spectrum disorders in humans and genes associated with social responsiveness in honeybees.

16. Rahman MM. Neurological effects of honey: current and future prospects. *Evidence Based Complementary and Alternative Medicine* 2014; 2014; Article 958721. DOI: 10.1155/2014/958721.

Note: The authors demonstrated that raw honey and honey polyphenols attenuated microglia-induced neuroinflammation. This is an excellent study from Bangladesh and Malaysia that comprehensively outlines the neuroprotective benefits of honey and its bioflavonoids – and the combating of microglia-induced neuroinflammation articulated in the later study by Palmieri (reference 18 below) – blockade of glutamine synthetase, the enzyme of cognition, communication and language.

17. Kanimozhi S, Subramanian P, Shanmugapriya S, Sathishkumar S. Role of bioflavonoid quercetin on Expression of Urea Cycle Enzymes, Astrocytic and Inflammatory Markers in Hyperammonaemia Rats. *Indian Journal of Clinical Biochemistry* 2017; 32(1): 68-73.
DOI: 10.1007/s12291-016-0575-8. PMID: 28149015

Note: This brilliant study from Annamalai University, Tamil Nadu, India, demonstrated anti-ammonia benefits of quercetin; the mechanism may be due to increased glutamine synthetase, the only enzyme in the human brain that controls ammonia levels. The authors noted that treatment with quercetin significantly enhanced the expression of glutamine synthetase. This historic study has secured only one citation in the PubMed library – a shocking indictment of western science.

18. Palmieri EM, Menga A, Lebrun A, et al. Blockade of Glutamine Synthetase Enhances Inflammatory Response in Microglial Cells. *Antioxidant & Redox Signaling* 2017; 26(8): 351-363. DOI: 10.1089/ars.2016.6715. PMID: 27758118

19. Chen S, Jiang H, Wu X, Fang J. Therapeutic Effects of Quercetin on Inflammation, Obesity, and Type 2 Diabetes. *Hindawi Mediators of Inflammation* 2016; 2016: 9340637. DOI: 10.1155/2016/9340637. PMID: 28003714

Note: This is an excellent study showing potent anti-inflammatory activity of quercetin in obesity and diabetes. Quercetin is a major and universal honey bioflavonoid.

20. Dhanya R, Arya AD, Nisha P, Jayamurthy P. Quercetin, a Lead Compound against Type 2 Diabetes Ameliorates Glucose Uptake via AMPK Pathway in Skeletal Muscle Cell Line. *Frontiers in Pharmacology* 2017; 8: 336. DOI: 10.3389/fphar.2017.00336. PMID: 28642704

Note: This is an excellent study on the effect of quercetin, a major honey bioflavonoid, on blood glucose control, from India and Pakistan. The authors showed that quercetin shared a similar mechanism with the anti-diabetic drug metformin, highlighting it as a promising compound for the management of type 2 diabetes. Quercetin cannot of course be patented though there have been filings for different combinations that include it.

21. Khan H, Ullah H, Aschner M, et al. Neuroprotective Effects of Quercetin in Alzheimer's Disease. *Biomolecules* 2020; 10(1): 59. DOI: 10.3390/biom10010059. PMID: 31905923

Note: This is an excellent review of the multiple neurological benefits of quercetin by a combined team from China, Pakistan, Turkey and America. The authors discovered that quercetin protects neurones by attenuating oxidative stress and neuroinflammation. The anti-Alzheimer's disease properties of quercetin include the inhibition of amyloid-beta aggregation and tau protein phosphorylation.

22. Alvarez-Arellano L, Salazar-Garcia M, Corona JC. Neuroprotective Effects of Quercetin in Pediatric Neurological Diseases. *Molecules* 2020; 25(23): 5597.
DOI: 10.3390/molecules25235597. PMID: 33260783

Note: The authors found quercetin was a suitable adjuvant for therapy against paediatric neurological diseases. The major pathways of sugar-induced neurodegeneration are oxidation of glutamine synthetase in microglial cells, followed by chronic inflammation and increased glutamate toxicity, followed by cell death of neurones. These neuropathological events are also induced by insulin resistance, hyperinsulinaemia and elevated glutamate toxicity. They are opposed by quercetin oestrogen signalling, quercetin protection against hyperinsulinism, quercetin protection from oxidation and quercetin protection against inflammation.

# References for Figures 1, 3, 4, 5 and 7

F1. Guyenet S. By 2606, the US Diet will be 100 Percent Sugar. *Whole Food Source* 18 February 2012. https://wholehealthsource. blogspot.com/2012/02/by-2606-us-diet-will-be-100-percent.html (accessed 24 April 2023)

F2. Valabhji J. Spotlight on diabetes. NHS-75 England. 20 April 2018. www.england.nhs.uk/blog/spotlight-on-diabetes/ (accessed 24 April 2023)

F3. Parikh NI, Pencina MJ, Wang TJ, et al. Increasing trends in incidence of overweight and obesity over 5 decades. *Am J Med* 2007; 120(3): 242-250.e2

F4. Khan M, Hashim MJ, King JK, et al. Epidemiology of type 2 diabetes. *J Epidemiol Global Health* 2020; 10(1): 107-111.

F5. Lin X, Xu Y, Pan X, et al. Global, regional and national burden and trend of diabetes in 195 countries and territories: an analysis from 1990 to 2025. *Sci Rep: J Pharmaeut Policy Prac* 2020; 10: 14790. DOI: org/10.1038/s41598-020-71908-9

F6. WHO. Diabetes Fact Sheet. 5 April 2023. World Health Organization.

F7. Li X, Feng X, Sun X, et al. Global, regional and national burden of Alzheimer's disease and other dementias 1990-2019. *Front Aging Neurosci* 2022; 14: 937486. DOI: 10.3389/fnagi.2022.937486. PMID 36299608

R8. CDC. Autism prevalence. 23 March 2023. Centers for Disease Control and Prevention, US. (Accessed 24 April 2023)

F9. Rivell A, Mattson MP. Intergenerational metabolic syndrome and neuronal network hyperexcitability in autism. *Trends Neurosci* 2019; 42(10): 709-726. DOI: 10.1016/j.tins.2019.08.006. PMID 31495451

# Glossary

**AGEs (advanced glycation end-products)** are proteins and fats (lipids) that have been exposed to excess circulating glucose. Sugar molecules are 'sticky' and if they attach to other circulating molecules, they damage them and render them non-functional. They are associated with physiological degenerative diseases, in particular diabetes, kidney disease and atherosclerosis. They are increasingly implicated in neurodegenerative conditions – obesity, type 2 diabetes, Alzheimer's disease and autism spectrum disorders.

**Amino acids** are the building blocks of proteins. All proteins are simple or complex combinations of amino acids, and there are 21 common to all life forms. Nine are 'essential' in the human diet in that we cannot make these for ourselves: valine, isoleucine, phenylalanine, tryptophan, threonine, histidine and lysine. Glutamine (see page 41) is not considered 'essential' but is one of six regarded as 'conditionally essential' meaning that their synthesis may be limited by disease or other circumstances. These are: arginine, cysteine, glutamine, glycine, proline and tyrosine.

**Apoptosis** is the scientific term for programmed (intentional) cell death. There are multiple events that may lead to cell death. A healthy human adult may lose up to 50 billion cells daily. In this book the focus is on neurodegenerative conditions that generate pathological apoptosis via excess sugar-driven loss of neurones – the result of oxidation/inflammation/glutamate excitotoxicity/calcium overload and mitochondrial depolarisation.

**Astrocytes,** also known as **astroglia** and simply 'glia', are special cells in the brain and spinal cord that are star shaped. They surround neurones and connect to the endothelial cells of the brain capillaries, thereby acting as a key component of the blood-brain barrier. They provide nutrients, energy and oxygen to the brain and house the brain's fuel pump – the enzyme glutamine synthetase.

**Benign ketosis** is a weight loss strategy whereby a very low level of carbohydrate consumptions triggers the use of ketones to fuel the brain. It was a strategy that allowed our hunter-gatherer ancestors to survive during starvation and famine when food/energy reserves were low. Body fat stores were raided to release ketones (small fat molecules) to fuel both brain and body. It has often been confused or associated (incorrectly) with ketoacidosis (particularly by health professionals), a dangerous condition.

**Bioflavonoids** are polyphenolic compounds widespread in the plant kingdom and consumed by humans in fruit and vegetables. They exert almost universally positive influence in all the pathways involving energy consumption, transport, partition, distribution and disposal, and therefore are being actively researched for potential benefits in late-modern human neurodegenerative diseases: obesity, type 2 diabetes, Alzheimer's disease and autism spectrum disorders. Honey contains around 30 of these principles, depending on the variety, and therefore is the perfect fuel to protect the brain from excess sugar-driven neurotoxicity and thereby advance human cognition, communication and language.

**Blood-brain barrier** is the term for the tight control on the movement of ions, molecules and cells into the brain that is exercised by the blood vessels that vascularise the central nervous system and work with glia to ensure neurones receive the right amount of energy, oxygen and nutrients.

**Cell surface receptors** are transmembrane receptors that are embedded in the membranes of biological cells. They act as signalling systems by binding to extracellular molecules, such as hormones, neurotransmitters, cytokine immune signals, growth factors and various nutrients, which alter internal cell metabolism and function. They include transmembrane proteins, glycoproteins and lipoproteins. They are targets in drug research whereby cell function may be modulated positively or negatively depending on the intended modification and the condition involved.

**Enzymes** are (usually complex) proteins that function as catalysts in the conversion of one biological molecule to another. Almost all metabolic reactions in the processing of foods – digestion, absorption, breakdown, transport, integration and disposal via biosynthesis and excretion – require enzymes to function. In this book much attention is paid to the ancient enzyme glutamine synthetase (which first appeared in the fossil record 3.8 billion years ago) that functions as the human brain's fuel pump: each conversion of excitotoxic glutamate to beneficial glutamine by glutamine synthetase pumps a glucose molecule from the circulation into the brain. It is the excess sugar-driven oxidative degradation of glutamine synthetase that defines the four sugar-sickness syndromes: obesity, type 2 diabetes, Alzheimer's disease and autism spectrum disorders.

**Epigenetics** is the study of alterations in gene expression that are heritable, and may cross from one generation to the other, but do not involve mutations or alterations in DNA sequences. It is a growing field of study – switching genes on or off may have healthy or unhealthy consequences. Diet is a major influence on epigenetic-modulated gene expression, exerting both positive and negative influence on health. Excess refined sugars are a recognised influence on negative epigenetic expression.

**Excitotoxicity:** Nerve cells are damaged or destroyed by neurotrans-mitters such as glutamate that are essential but become dangerously high resulting in excessive stimulation of receptors.

**Free radicals** are molecules that are unstable and likely to react with other molecules because they contain an unpaired electron.

**Gene expression** is the process by which a gene is switched on in a cell to make proteins. Excess refined sugars negatively influence gene expression in metabolic (energy) pathways. Honey does the opposite.

**Glia/glial cells** are the critical cells supporting neurones in the brain and peripheral nervous systems. They provide neurones with energy, water, oxygen and nutrients that enable neurones to survive and function. They also provide structural support which, until recently, was thought to be their only function (the word 'glia' is derived from the Greek for 'glue'). They house the human brain's fuel pump – the enzyme glutamine synthetase. The breakdown of energy regulation in glia is the primary driving force in all sugar sickness syndromes.

**Gluconeogenesis** is the process of manufacturing glucose from non-carbohydrate sources when glucose reserves are low, mainly from muscle proteins. The process occurs during famine and starvation so that the brain is sufficiently provisioned. The liver is the major site of gluconeogenesis. However, late-modern humans consuming excess sugar paradoxically and chronically activate this process because the sugar suppression of the enzyme glutamine synthetase deprives the brain of energy and places this organ in a semi-starvation state; this activates gluconeogenesis and the new glucose synthesised and released simply adds to the problem of excessively high blood sugar, a vicious negative cycle. Muscles are degraded and this explains why it is so difficult for overweight and obese persons to exercise. The process requires release of stress hormones. Endurance athletes who fail to fuel optimally also lose muscle via gluconeogenesis and the catabolism (breakdown) of muscle protein driven by stress hormones leads to many unhealthy outcomes.

**Glutamate** (also known as **glutamic acid**) is the major excitatory neurotransmitter at almost all synapses in the human central nervous system (CNS) and peripheral nervous system (PNS). Glutamate functions as both the hunger signal in the human brain and as the 'spark plug' in firing the brain's engine, by activating the enzyme glutamine synthetase to convert it to beneficial glutamine, a process that pumps glucose into the brain. Late-modern humans consuming excess sugar suffer from excess glutamate in the central nervous system, and thereby a deficiency of glutamine; this picture is a major biomarker for impaired glutamine synthetase.

**Glutamine** is the most abundant free amino acid in the human circulation. It is regarded as non-essential (meaning that it may be synthesised in the human body and therefore not required in the human diet). However, it is often referred to as 'conditionally essential' when demand is increased during stressful conditions such as infections. Glutamine is widely available in proteins in a healthy human diet, although it is highly unstable, and a significant portion is used by the gut and immune system as fuel. In late-modern humans consuming excess sugar, the enzyme glutamine synthetase is oxidatively suppressed and compromised, meaning that glutamine becomes more essential than non-essential. This is the key to each of the sugar sickness syndromes, whereby glutamine becomes deficient – a finding from long-Covid-induced viral hyperglycaemia and characterised by chronic glutamine deficiency in the brain.

**Glutamatergic pathway:** This consists of neural pathways where synapses between neurones use the neurotransmitter glutamate and postsynaptic receptors are specifically sensitive to glutamate. If the enzyme glutamine synthetase in glia functions healthily, and the glutamate/glutamine ratio is balanced, the glutamatergic pathway functions optimally.

**Glutamate/glutamine (G/G) cycle:** This cycle is one of the oldest and most significant cycles in human metabolism. Glutamate, the hunger and excitotoxic signal in energy metabolism in the brain, is converted to beneficial glutamine in glia; each cycle transfers a glucose molecule into the brain, providing it with the energy it needs. Nitrogen is added to glutamate to form glutamine thereby using free nitrogen and preventing build-up of toxic ammonia. If the cycle is impaired, toxic build-up of glutamate in synapses causes a cascade of negative influences that result in metabolic diseases, obesity, type 2 diabetes, Alzheimer's disease and autism spectrum disorders.

**Glutamine synthetase** is the enzyme that I describe in this book as the brain's fuel pump. The glutamine synthetase gene is one of the oldest functioning genes in the history of evolution (3.8 billion years). Prior to and beyond the evolution of multicellular organisms around 2 billion years ago, this enzyme was involved in nitrogen metabolism. From around 500 million years ago, when the primitive nervous systems first appeared, it was co-opted as the fuel pump to maintain energy supply into the evolving and increasingly complex nervous systems of living organisms. In humans this enzyme converts excitotoxic glutamate (the brain's hunger signal) to beneficial glutamine, and each turn of the cycle pumps a glucose molecule into a glial cell that supplies a neurone with energy, oxygen and other nutrients. In this sense glutamine synthetase is the enzyme of cognition, communication and language, each of which is compromised if the enzyme is impaired.

**Glutathione** is an ancient antioxidant in plants, animals, fungi and bacteria. It is synthesised from the amino acids, glycine, cysteine and glutamic acid (glutamate). It protects cells from reactive oxygen species, free radicals, and other oxidative molecules such as heavy metals. In humans it is mostly synthesised in the liver, and functions as the most significant antioxidant in body and brain.

**Glycaemia** is a term for the presence of glucose in the human circulation. High blood glucose concentration is hyperglycaemia. Low blood glucose concentration is hypoglycaemia.

**Glycaemic index (GI)** is a way to measure the impact of foods that contain carbohydrates on blood sugar levels, on a scale of 0 (zero impact) to 100 (pure glucose). Below 55 is regarded as a relatively low GI.

**Hormones** are signalling molecules (chemical messengers) that are delivered from glands in the body via the circulation to various organs and tissues, affecting multiple pathways that maintain homeostasis (balance). They affect every aspect of prenatal physical and neurological development, growth, reproduction and ageing. These include digestion, metabolism, respiration, sensory perception, sleep/circadian rhythm, excretion, lactation, stress induction, movement, locomotion and mood.

**Hyperglycaemia** is a condition in which excess levels of glucose in the bloodstream cause multiple pathological processes in body and brain. The normal and healthy level of blood glucose is up to 100 mg/decilitre – that is, per 100 mg/100 ml. Alternatively, this can be measured in millimoles per litre, with the normal range being 4.0 to 5.9 mmol/l. Above 126 mg/100 ml is considered to be diabetic. If not quickly resolved, chronic hyperglycaemia is dangerous, negatively influencing every cell in the human body. In this book I show how hyperglycaemia (caused by overconsumption of refined carbohydrates and sugars, or by environmental factors such as infection and urban air pollution) is the major influence in obesity, type 2 diabetes, Alzheimer's disease and autism spectrum disorders.

**Hyperinsulinaemia** is the term to describe when the level of insulin in the bloodstream is higher than is healthy, generally as a result of insulin resistance.

**Hyperinsulinism:** Usually a genetic disorder in which the pancreas secretes too much insulin resulting in low blood sugar (hypoglycaemia); this can also be caused by pancreatic tumours (insulinomas).

**Hyperperfusion** is the term for abnormally increased blood flow to an organ, and in this book, specifically to the brain. It usually refers to a condition whereby cerebral blood flow is dysregulated due to dilation of the blood vessels that supply the brain. In severe cases it may cause seizures or coma.

**Hypoglycaemia** is the term for a rapid fall in blood glucose concentration, below 70 mg/decilitre (100 ml). It is a very dangerous condition, resulting if not quickly resolved in confusion, fatigue, sweating, shakes, hunger, rapid heart rate, loss of consciousness, coma and eventually death. The most common cause globally is that of antidiabetic drugs, including insulin, whereby the dose is misjudged relative to eating and an episode follows. The condition refers to physiological hypoglycaemia. However, much neglected is chronic cerebral hypoglycaemia caused not by systemically low blood glucose, but by high blood glucose (hyperglycaemia). This results in oxidative degradation of glutamine synthetase, the human brain's fuel pump, and is the major driving force in the neurodegenerative conditions obesity, type 2 diabetes, Alzheimer's disease and autism spectrum disorders.

**Hypoperfusion** is a condition of low blood flow, and is usually caused by low blood pressure, heart failure or loss of blood volume. Symptoms include light-headedness, dizziness, headache, nausea, fatigue and shortness of breath. In acute situations it is described as 'shock' characterised by low oxygen delivery to tissues. Signs include low blood pressure, tachypnoea (rapid and shallow breathing), cool and clammy skin, agitation and impaired mental status. In the sugar sickness syndromes the brain is dehydrated due to hyperglycaemia blocking the aquaporin channels (cross-cell membrane proteins involved in water transfer) and doubly so due to loss of osmotic transfer of water (less cerebral glucose). Paradoxically in Long-Covid along with glutamine deficiency there is increased water accumulation due to overproduction of hyaluranon, which traps water in the cellular matrix – a double blow – too little water combined with trapped and unusable water. In the brain the water is trapped in the vital structural hyaluranon-rich extracellular matrix and adds to the dehydration.

**Hypoxia** is a condition in which the body is deprived of oxygen and may be global or specific to one tissue or organ. It is a well recognised feature of high altitude and underwater diving. Severe hypoxia is extremely dangerous, causing confusion, breathlessness, slow heart rate, low blood pressure and heart failure, leading to coma and death. Hyperglycaemia is a recognised cause of hypoxia in cells. It blocks the aquaporin channels that facilitate oxygen transfer. In the brain hyperglycaemia blocks oxygen transfer into glia, a process that suppresses glutamine synthetase, and the brain is deprived of both oxygen and glucose (energy). Cerebral hypoxia is a feature of the four sugar sickness syndromes.

**Inflammation** is the reaction of the body to invasion by pathogens, infective or otherwise, when the protective immune system is activated in response. Heat is induced as part of the process (to kill infective pathogens), and pain is involved – also a protective measure – with redness, swelling of tissue and loss of function. Children often suffer from the unpleasant symptoms due to cuts, scratches and boils. Inflammation is most often associated with hay fever and other allergies, dental disease, atherosclerosis and osteoarthritis. Anti-inflammatory drugs are often prescribed. Inflammation of the brain is usually chronic and secondary to oxidation due to excess glucose in the circulation, which sets off an inflammatory cascade in brain microglia (immune cells) – a major feature of all metabolic (energy dysregulation) diseases. Neurones and synapses are engulfed leading to impaired cognition.

**Insulin** is a hormone that is produced by specialised beta cells in the pancreas. Its primary role is that of an anabolic (building) hormone. It regulates carbohydrate, fat and protein metabolism. Although its roles are many, it is most commonly associated with glucose metabolism, whereby it promotes glucose uptake into cells, in particular liver, muscle and fat (adipose) cells. Insulin is released by the pancreas in response to glucose and proteins, not to fats. However, insulin does influence fat regulation by promoting conversion of glucose to fats and storing them in fat cells. Among its many roles are: stimulating glucose uptake by cells and tissues, thereby reducing blood glucose concentration; increasing fat synthesis; decreasing lipolysis (release of fats from stores); increasing storage of glucose as glycogen in liver and muscle cells; reducing the release of glucose from the liver; reducing gluconeogenesis (manufacture of glucose from protein); and decreasing the breakdown of muscle proteins to make glucose to promote gluconeogenesis. Less well recognised is its role in the brain where it is synthesised by specialised neurones and is directly involved in memory and cognition. Insulin functions as the cerebral fuel governor whereby it regulates the fuel pump, glutamine synthetase, which in turn counter-regulates insulin. Cerebral insulin resistance, also known as central insulin resistance, is now a recognised negative influence on brain energy regulation, and a major feature of the excess-sugar-driven neurodegenerative conditions, obesity, type 2 diabetes, Alzheimer's disease and autism spectrum disorders. These conditions are now being recognised as a form of 'type 3 diabetes'.

**Insulin resistance** is a pathological condition whereby cells increasingly fail to respond to the hormone insulin, or the insulin receptors are downgraded in response to excess production of insulin (hyperinsulinaemia). Late-modern (post 1970s) humans are chronically prone to hyperinsulinaemia due to excess consumption of refined sugars and carbohydrates.

**Keto-adaptation** is the process of replacing glucose as the primary fuel for the body and brain with ketones – small fat molecules. It is essentially a state of switching fuels from carbohydrates to fats.

**Ketogenic diet:** This is a high-fat/adequate-protein/low-carbohydrate diet whereby the primary fuel of body and brain is fat/ketones.

**Ketoacidosis** is a dysregulated energy (metabolic) state caused by uncontrolled production of ketones, a dangerous acidic alteration of the acid/base (pH) balance in the body, most often associated with diabetes, that occurs when there is insufficient insulin to allow blood glucose into cells for energy.

**Ketosis** is the production of ketones, small fat molecules that may act as fuel for body and brain. It occurs when glucose reserves are low, and helps maintain essential energy levels in the brain.

**Metabolic syndrome** is a complex condition consisting of obesity, high blood pressure, excess blood glucose levels, increased circulating fats and low levels of high-density lipoproteins. It is associated with increased risk of cardiovascular disease. Only 6.8% of Americans have healthy cardiometabolic syndrome suggesting that 93.2% have metabolic syndrome. The various biomarkers in this condition are indicative of insulin resistance/hyperinsulinaemia and consequent neurodegenerative conditions.

**Microglia** are specialised glia (support cells), in the brain and peripheral nervous system. They function as the nervous system's immune cells. They remain in a deactivated state until a threat appears in the nervous system that may be infective, toxic or other. They migrate to the site of injury and enter a state of high activation, releasing immune factors to attack, neutralise and expel such threats. In the microglia the enzyme glutamine synthetase is the key immune regulator; oxidative degradation of this enzyme activates an inflammatory cascade that engulfs neurones and synapses. Each of the sugar sickness syndromes is associated with chronic overactivation of microglia, the major driving force of neurodegeneration.

**Necrosis** is a form of cell injury that may result in the apoptosis (see page 229) of the cell when subject to attack by any pathogen, infective or other. Cell death by apoptosis may remove injured cells that pose a threat, but necrosis is more lethal and dangerous.

**Neurones** are electrically excitable brain cells that communicate with each other and other cells by propagating electrical signals along an axon and between cells via synaptic gaps, that continue the information signalling using neurotransmitters that cross the synapse and transmit the signal by attaching to receptors on the post synaptic neurone.

Neurones are the major signalling cells in the central nervous system (brain and spinal cord) and the peripheral nervous system, connecting the brain to the various organs, limbs and tissues that are under the control of the brain, the central processor.

**Neurotransmitters** are signalling molecules secreted by neurones to enable electrical signals to cross the synaptic gaps between cells, by binding to receptors. Neurotransmitters are usually very simple molecules, synthesised from amino acids. The major neurotransmitter referenced in this book is glutamate but others include serotonin, dopamine and acetylcholine.

**Nocturnal fast:** This is a period of semi-starvation when the brain is at risk of entering stress physiology. The liver glycogen store is very small (around 75-100 grams if optimally fuelled). This is the only reserve energy store available to provision the brain during the nocturnal fast. However, the liver at rest releases around 10 grams of glucose per hour – 6.5 grams to the brain and 3.5 grams to the kidneys and red blood cells. From an early evening meal around 6:00-7:00 pm there is simply not enough brain fuel to last for the 12 hours until breakfast. The brain activates gluconeogenesis to improve its fuel reserve, but that is a problem because liver insulin resistance inhibits this process. Nocturnal metabolic stress inhibits memory formation and consolidation, and cognition is compromised. Late-modern humans are experiencing an epidemic of stress-induced sleeplessness and should therefore consider refuelling the liver glycogen store prior to sleep. Honey is the ideal food for this purpose.

**Oxidation** of any biologically active molecule involves loss of electrons. All molecules are vulnerable to oxidation, including oxygen itself. Living entities – animals, plants and organisms – are all subject to oxidation and must develop antioxidant systems as a survival strategy. Every living cell oxidises fuel to release the energy required to survive and function and that process is the most toxic threat against call survival. In humans, oxidative degradation of sugars, fats and proteins is profoundly damaging. In this book oxidative degradation of the enzyme glutamine synthetase in brain glia and microglia, leading to inflammation in the microglia, is the initiating and driving force of the neurodegenerative conditions, obesity, type 2 diabetes, Alzheimer's disease and autism spectrum disorders.

**Oxygen species** are unstable, oxygen-containing molecules that are highly reactive with other molecules – free radicals – and therefore may cause damage to DNA, RNA and whole cells.

**Partition** is the division of available energy between the parts of a multicellular organism needing it. When foods are ingested, they are broken down in the gut and enter the circulation, mainly through the liver. In terms of energy provision, the energy-containing molecules are divided between (partitioned into) various organs and tissues. The healthy human brain, which has no significant energy store, always takes priority, and has an energy pumping system that ensures its supply is exquisitely regulated to meet immediate demand, but not oversupply it, which is highly dangerous. Partition in this case is critical to brain survival. Because the regulation process breaks down in modern sugar-driven energy dysregulation diseases, these are characterised by chronic brain energy deficiency and chronic body energy surfeit.

**Polyphenols** are naturally occurring organic molecules that are structurally diverse and are abundant in plants, including many of the plants that are included in the human diet, in particular in fruit and vegetables. Polyphenols and their major group, bioflavonoids, are known to counter many of the pathological systems that appear in modern degenerative diseases, and significantly in neurodegenerative conditions. Polyphenols seem to have evolved from ancient algae and were key to survival in the migration onto the land of early plant species some 500 million years ago. They were then critical in the coevolution of honeybees with flowering plants (from 100 million years ago). They enable the honeybee to process colossal quantities of sugar during flight and yet maintain excellent foraging and pollination cognition.

**Pyroptosis** is the term for inflammatory cell death due to overheating. When microglia are activated due to any brain insult, including sugar-driven oxidative suppression of glutamine synthetase, an inflammatory cascade is activated in these cells that engulfs and consumes neurones. Essentially this is a form of cooking and digesting the human brain.

**Quercetin** is a plant flavonoid found in fruit, vegetables, seeds and some grains. It is also found in all varieties of honey and acts as an antioxidant and anti-inflammatory, and is neuroprotective. It is one of many bioflavonoids in honey, all of which are similarly neuroprotective. Indeed, quercetin and the other bioflavonoids in honey protect against all the major damage that refined sugars inflict on the human brain, including oxidation, inflammation, impaired glutamine synthetase, excess excitotoxic glutamate, glutamine deficiency, hypoxia, cerebral glucose energy deficiency, cerebral dehydration and hyperglycaemia. Quercetin and the other bioflavonoids in honey offer an alternative sweetener in foods and drinks that is both antidiabetic and neuroprotective.

**Sensory perception disorder**, also known as **sensory processing disorder** is the failure to perceive and respond to sensory information both from the environment and internally and can be associated with being overly sensitive as well as under sensitive to stimuli. It is a global condition with impaired visual (sight), olfactory (smell), auditory (hearing), gustatory (taste) and tactile (touch) information processing, including the internal senses. It is most often associated with autism spectrum disorders and attention-deficit hyperactivity disorder. However, it extends way beyond these conditions and affects around 15% of elementary school children. This is deeply alarming and, although the condition falls beneath the radar of the health institutions, health professionals, government and the public, it should be recognised as perhaps the major threat to future cognition. We know that no information may enter the human nervous system without being coupled with the expensive energy required to integrate and encode it, the major function of the enzyme glutamine synthetase. We also know that glutamine synthetase is degraded in the brain and peripheral nervous system glia via excess circulating glucose. We recognise that sensory processing is impaired in each of the sugar sickness syndromes. We may therefore infer that if a child exits the womb free of an autism spectrum disorder, he or she may then be subject to sugar-induced sensory processing disorder, a form of **postnatal autism** that threatens the child's future as a cognitively competent individual.

**Stress:** In humans, stress may be physiological or psychological. It is the human response to a real or perceived threat. Two major hormones, adrenaline and cortisol, are mobilised – adrenaline via the autonomic nervous system and cortisol via the hypothalamus-pituitary-axis. These hormones are popularly described as fight-or-flight hormones. They are released during a fight-or-flight episode such as a predator threat, but that description fails to account for the most frequent release of these hormones. They are essentially neuroprotective, shielding the brain from loss of energy supply. Our response to any threatening situation involving the flight response uses up circulating blood glucose and poses a challenge to the brain, which has no significant fuel store. If the brain is in danger of running out of fuel, this selfish organ will bring the flight to a stop (athletes 'bonk'/collapse). The brain, protected within the skull, will survive somewhat longer than the body in the case of an attack. In late-modern humans consuming excess sugar, the brain is chronically under threat from loss of energy supply due to sugar-driven suppression of its fuel pump – glutamine synthetase. Therefore, the brain is chronically compelled to activate the stress response in the absence of a physical or other threat.

**Sugar sickness syndromes** is the collective term I use throughout this book to describe the four neurodegenerative conditions caused by excess consumption of refined carbohydrates and sugars.

**Synapses** are gaps between nerve cells (neurones) that enable signalling to be transmitted from a pre-synaptic neurone to a post-synaptic neurone via neurotransmitters (chemical messengers). The inclusion of synapses that control neurotransmission is a highly sophisticated system that regulates the brain and nervous system signalling such that excess signalling is prevented by increased uptake and removal of a transmitter if the situation requires it. For instance, serotonin, a hormone and neurotransmitter with many functions in the body, is involved in regulation of cognition, mood, appetite and sleep. Depression is a condition that may be modified positively in some people by serotonin reuptake inhibitors which inhibit the clearance of serotonin from synapses, thereby increasing serotonin signalling. Prozac is the most famous brand. There are many neurotransmitters in the human brain; around 100 have been identified. Glutamate is a major neurotransmitter and functions to regulate energy metabolism in the brain and nervous system.

**Urban hyperglycaemia** (also known as **urban diabetes**) is driven by insulin resistance – the result of urban air pollution that drives up blood glucose concentrations. It is increasingly recognised as a cause of obesity, type 2 diabetes, Alzheimer's disease and autism spectrum disorders.

**Viral hyperglycaemia (or viral diabetes)** is the overly high blood sugar level that accompanies many viral infections, including most recently Covid-19.

# Index

*Bold page references indicate glossary definitions. 'rn' after a page number indicates a reference note providing significant additional information.

245

---

*Bold page references indicate glossary definitions. 'rn' after a page number indicates a reference note providing significant additional information.

# Index

---

*Bold page references indicate glossary definitions. 'rn' after a page number indicates a reference note providing significant additional information.

*Bold page references indicate glossary definitions. 'rn' after a page number indicates a reference note providing significant additional information.

# Index

*Bold page references indicate glossary definitions. 'rn' after a page number
indicates a reference note providing significant additional information.

---

*Bold page references indicate glossary definitions. 'rn' after a page number indicates a reference note providing significant additional information.